The Carb Party DIET

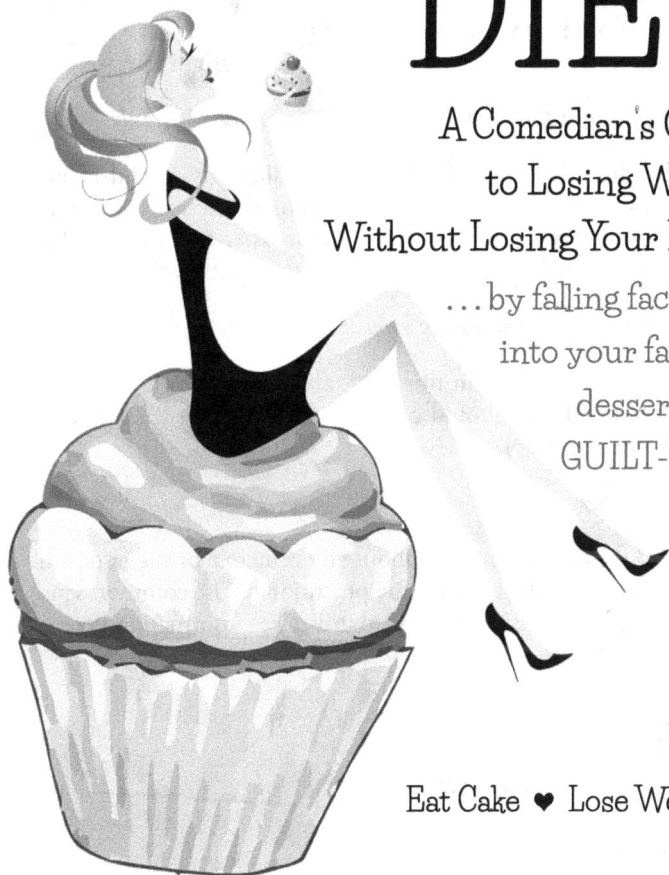

A Comedian's Guide
to Losing Weight
Without Losing Your Mind
...by falling face-first
into your favorite
dessert tray,
GUILT-FREE

Eat Cake ♥ Lose Weight

Laura Bartlett & Hannah Sinclair

The Carb Party Diet: A Comedian's Guide to Losing Weight Without Losing Your Mind . . . by falling face-first into your favorite dessert tray, GUILT-FREE

Bartlett-Sinclair Publications © 2016

The information in this book is for informational purposes only.

The reader should not use this book as medical advice and its authors are not, nor do they claim to be, licensed physicians. The information in this book is based on personal experiences and understanding of the available research at the date of publication.

This book is for healthy adults and not intended for children.

The principles found within this book are intended for adults only over the age of 21. You should consult with your physician to confirm individual appropriateness.

Use Common Sense.

If you need further clarification about any principle or suggestion in this book, ask a qualified health care practitioner. Use common sense to make your best decision on how to utilize the information herein.

Print ISBN: 978-0-99723-740-5

eBook ISBN: 978-0-99723-741-2

CarbPartyDiet.com

CONTENTS

INTRODUCTION

Do you want a deliciously simple way to lose stubborn body fat? Then this is the book for you! Let's face it—most women would rather give up their right kidney than give up carbs forever. Good news: you don't have to. *The Carb Party Diet* is a fat-loss system created specifically for women, by women! You'll learn how to *overeat* "bad" foods to lose belly fat (. . . crazy, but true). You'll never again diet alone but instead have fun doing it with your girlfriends! See, *The Carb Party Diet* believes that "it takes a village . . . to lose a pound!" In other words, weight-loss success is directly related to a close-knit community of supportive, like-minded girlfriends, a sort of Ya-Ya sisterhood of women. Besides, what woman doesn't like a Girls' Night Out?!

But can you really eat cookies, cake and ice cream to lose weight? The answer is an enthusiastic YES! A Carb Party isn't merely permitted but is *necessary* to keep your leptin levels high. It's fun, effective, and delicious to follow. It's based on a plethora of cutting-edge medical research and science related to hormone rebalancing.

Truth is, you too could have discovered this on your own—but it would have been exhausting and time consuming to wade through unscrupulous diet industry advertising and marketing B.S., and mounds of medical research. That's why we did it for you. We created this easy-to-follow, step-by-step guide to forever liberate you from diet scams and fads. You'll finally understand how to control carbs instead of carbs controlling you. As a result, it'll transform your old metabolism into a 24/7 fat-burning machine. Forget about needing fancy online nutrition calculators and being a slave to "personal coaching programs." It's all here. You'll understand which ordinary foods to eat and when to eat them, to repair and improve your leptin and insulin sensitivity so you can lose fat and keep it off. You'll finally learn the truth about eating fat (prepare to be surprised!). You'll discover how to eat cookies (rather than eliminate them forever) to supercharge your metabolism, kill cravings, and never yo-yo diet again. It's Hannah's and Laura's hope that this book will create a grassroots movement to reverse the obesity epidemic and get women healthy again.

1

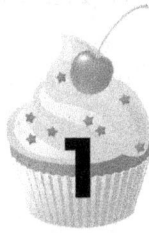

Hannah's Story

Been There, Done That, Got the Frustration to Prove It

"My life hasn't always been a fun, food-frenzy party. Adolescence and those awkward teenage years were brutal. Many mistakes were made. Many tears were shed. Then the weight-loss light bulb came on."

**—Hannah Sinclair,
fed-up dieter, experimenter extraordinaire**

My First Bikini

My chubby stomach was perpetually five shades lighter than my legs, a result of being shielded for 14 years behind a stretched wall of swimsuit spandex, otherwise known as the modest one-piece bathing suit.

I remember mustering up the courage to ask my mom, "Do you think maybe *now* I can wear a bikini?"

Excited by the possibility of some rare mother-daughter bonding, she pulled me aside and then, leaning toward her dresser drawers, she suggested, "Maybe you could wear one of *my* bikinis."

I shrugged: "OK, but it's probably not going to fit." Mom proceeded to rifle through her drawers.

During the flurry of sorting and sifting, she grabbed one of the most faded floral Goodwill-worthy two-piece suits in the drawer and flung it toward me. "Try this."

I shuffled off to a private corner of her room, crouched down, and began changing.

My mom, a huge fan of reality TV, anxiously anticipated the big reveal.

"Let me see!" she squealed.

The straps disappeared into my chubby shoulders.

"What the crap?" I thought. "When did they start making bikinis with dental floss?"

"Turn around," Mom blurted.

I did a quick 180 and let out a long, depressed sigh.

After scanning my body up and down several times, Mom conceded: "You know . . . we can always try to find you a cute tankini."

In my insecure mind, my mom's words screamed, "You know what you need? A full-length scuba suit!! BAHAHAHAHAHA!!"

It was at that moment, standing half naked in Mom's bedroom, it occurred to me: "I'm a fat girl."

My First Day of High School

It was the first day of school, and I have to admit, I was feeling pretty good. I was wearing a white, V-neck T-shirt, blue jeans and Keds. Pushing fashion boundaries, I sported a black plastic headband with a huge red, floppy flower.

Mom and I waited in the car for my brother Aaron.

Worried that we'd be late for school, Mom laid on the horn. Aaron locked the front door and leisurely made his way toward the car. "Move," he grunted. I slid over and did a double take. "WTF," I thought. Aaron had copied my "first day outfit" down to the sneakers. The only thing missing was a huge red flower.

As much as I wanted to argue that he needed to go back inside and change, it wasn't worth the strife. I had to pick my battles carefully. The last thing I wanted was to walk into school alone.

Somehow, despite being a geeky theater kid who wrestled, he had miraculously managed to successfully navigate the social land mines of high school unscathed.

In my mind, this automatically earned him "expert" status. His friends called him "Rubber Band Man." Mostly because of his superior flexibility and size: he was double-jointed and 93 pounds soaking wet.

But what didn't help him get dates more than paid off on the wrestling mat. His long and lanky body made him impossible to pin down.

As we walked around the back of the school, Aaron mumbled, "I need to talk to Coach." I followed instinctively to delay our separation.

Girls wrestling? Yep, it's really a thing . . .

As we entered the wrestling workout room, I became puzzled by what I saw.

"Who are *these* girls?" They looked nothing like I imagined female wrestlers to look.

Most had makeup on and were wearing skirts. They were even laughing and joking around.

"Hey Aaron, who's this?" one of the girls yelled. In a monotone voice, he answered, "This is my sister, Hannah." "Oh my gosh, she's so pretty!" another squealed and began playing with my long, naturally curly hair.

Weird boundary issues aside, I liked it. The positive attention made me feel accepted. I no longer needed Aaron as my crutch, and could do this thing called high school after all. I found my tribe.

The next morning, Mom drove us to Chick-fil-A for breakfast.

"I'll take a 20-piece chicken mini platter, a gallon of sweet tea and three large cups of ice," she screamed into the drive-thru speaker. It didn't take Aaron and me long to gobble down the entire order.

Soon, we were brushing the crumbs off our laps and making our way across the school campus into our first day of wrestling practice.

What a difference 24 hours made. A military cadence saturated the wrestling teams' mat room.

Shorts and high-laced wrestling shoes replaced skirts and heels. I was a wrestling newbie. I didn't really know what to expect. My only reference to wrestling was watching WWE on TV and wrestling my little brothers for the TV remote control.

I stood across the mat from one of best girl wrestlers in the state of Texas and prepared to improvise.

"BREEEEP," the coach's whistle blew. Fear and panic shot through my body. My teammate immediately began to drum my noggin with patronizing short finger jabs . . . a feeling I imagined my little brothers must have felt as I teased them, holding them at arm's length.

Then my sparring partner lunged toward my torso and took me down. My legs, tangled and unbalanced, quickly toppled. My head hit the floor with a resounding *whack*.

Instinctively, I rolled on my stomach and tried to crawl to safety. Seconds later, her body weight pressed into my lower back and my face nose-dived into the vinyl mat. Every breath was a struggle.

I quickly learned wrestling was very physically and mentally demanding. It was controlled chaos, and I loved every minute of it.

When we weren't working on wrestling techniques, coach had us doing crazy conditioning workouts like flipping truck tires. One particularly inventive workout was called the "Farm Girl," and required carrying five-gallon water buckets between two horse troughs.

It was like CrossFit on crack.

After winning a few tournaments, I finally felt and acted like a wrestler. I carried myself differently. I stood taller, shoulders back, with confidence in every step.

Any insecurity I still had was revealed during the weekly weigh-ins. I had chubby thighs and a spare-tire belly. I basically looked like a new mom struggling to lose that last 10 to 15 pounds of "baby fat."

My lower body was thick and bottom heavy. This was a significant advantage on the wrestling mat but not so much in a department store fitting room. My shape was so unique it didn't fall into the usual shape descriptors of pear, apple, etc.

Nope, more like bowling pin.

My Sophomore Year of High School

My siblings and I were "free range" and "corn fed." In addition to a childhood full of fun and outdoor adventures, it also contained breakfast pastries, peanut butter sandwiches, casseroles and after-school snacks.

Not unlike the diet of most teenagers across America.

I think I was subconsciously drawn to the sport of wrestling for its obsession with scales. Unlike any other high school sport, wrestling required weekly weigh-ins. I couldn't go over a certain fighting weight or I'd be disqualified from competition.

Over and over again, I had 24 hours to lose three pounds and a lifetime to deal with the OCD side-effects.

Honestly, everything I knew about "weight loss" came from watching TV talk shows and reading women's magazines.

Coach had his own weird diet tricks. He had us stand on a scale holding a sandwich. If we were over our fight weight, we were told to cut our sandwich in half and reweigh. Still too heavy? "Cut it again," he'd say. Whatever was left in your hand was what you were allowed to eat, often a fraction of the original.

Looking back, I can't believe I fell for such crazy advice. Applying the same logic, I should have eaten a steady diet of cotton candy, or foods just as light.

And when typical diets failed us, crazy wrestler hacks prevailed. It was perfectly normal to see girls on the wrestling team bundled up in layer after layer of clothing and spitting like camels into empty water bottles.

Our hope was that each lost millimeter of sweat or saliva would shift the scales in a positive direction.

One wrestler even cut her beautiful long hair. Unfortunately, she not only didn't make weight, but she was stuck with a really unflattering "mom bob."

Imagine a women's prison shower scene . . . yep, that's pretty close to what a weekly weigh-in looked like: naked girls of all sizes and ethnicities standing in long single-file lines waiting to be weighed. It was scary and humiliating.

Avoiding eye contact, I stared at a tramp stamp in front of me and thought, "How did I get here?" Just two years earlier, I was that insecure 14-year-old, crouching in Mom's bedroom trying on my first gently used bikini.

"NEXT!" barked the weigh-in lady.

It was my moment of truth. My bare feet stepped onto the cold scale. In a vain attempt, I sucked in my stomach and held my breath. After what felt like an eternity, I got the answer needed. "You're good to go!"

Making weight was an act of sheer will and luck.

My mom was a serial dieter. Being the only girl in the family, I was her accomplice. We tried every fad or trendy diet that promised quick results.

Whenever she had a few pounds to lose, she'd break out the chocolate SlimFast. When she got bored of chocolate shakes, she'd turn to the South Beach Diet.

So basically, I grew up understanding the definition of "diet" to mean "meal replacement" or "meal supplementation." I was clueless as to how they worked.

I chugged smoothies and hoped for the best.

My goal was to become a national wrestling champion, and I wasn't going to allow anything to get in the way. I considered abusing my body with metabolism-wrecking weight-loss methods, though not healthy, acceptable collateral damage.

We had been sparring for over an hour to get ready for one of the most important matches in the state of Texas.

The mat room's air was thick with evaporating sweat, yet unbearably hot at the same time. "WTF, why is it so damn hot?!" Coach had once again tricked the heater into believing it was minus 15 degrees by placing ice packs on the thermostat. The temperature soared somewhere between 80 degrees and Satan's butt crack.

Exhausted and unable to hear Coach's whistle, it happened. My sparring partner lunged toward me. Within seconds I was weightless. My body slammed into the mat, displacing a pool of sweat. The next thing I knew, I heard a loud *pop* and a lightning bolt of pain shot through my arm. Gripping my shoulder, I knew I was done.

My wrestling career was over.

My Junior Year of High School

Surgery was a blur, a combination of general anesthesia and pain meds. Doctors had to shave down multiple bone spurs and repair a torn bicep tendon.

For several months I was immobile and unable to do anything for myself. I felt like a two-year-old. My mom had to help me with everything, including personal hygiene.

The only upside to being physically limited was that I had a lot of time and few distractions. I decided to use my recovery time to focus on what I thought were healthier eating choices.

I replaced candy bars with protein bars, fast food with low-fat frozen meals, Pop-Tarts with peanut butter-smeared rice cakes. I replaced Cocoa Krispies with Mini-Wheats, sweet tea with fruit juice, and potato chips with trail mix.

My Senior Year of High School

Surprisingly, my eating habits stuck. For the remainder of high school, I continued to consciously eat what I believed was "healthier." If a food wasn't labeled "low fat," "less sugar," "no added sugar," "whole grain" or "organic," I didn't eat it.

Somehow, despite eating differently for two straight years, I was still fat, but even worse: I was constantly getting sick. I managed to catch every virus that was circulating. My immune system was shot. A cold turned into bronchitis.

After High School

Eighteen years old and sick, I finally scheduled a doctor's appointment.

As I waited to be seen, my index and middle fingers were pressed into the sides of my stuffy head. "Hannah?" the nurse interrupted.

I stood up and followed the nurse into the cold examination room.

I nervously kicked my legs back and forth, rustling the white butcher paper under my butt.

I stared at a Basal Metabolic Index (BMI) chart of a chunky pre-teen girl in an unflattering, purple one-piece swimsuit. The irony wasn't lost on me. A few years earlier, I *was* that girl.

"We got your blood work back," the doctor informed me. "And there are some things we need to discuss." In the next few minutes she explained that I was on a collision course toward diabetes, high cholesterol and other "old people" problems.

To add insult to injury, I was still fat. It was *déjà vu* . . .

Desperate and Dieting

Eager for a quick fix, I began trying every diet I knew. Nothing was off the table: fasting, calorie counting, vegetable juicing, South Beach Diet, SlimFast shakes, Special K Diet . . . you name it, I did it.

I read somewhere that apple cider vinegar was good for fat loss, so I began every morning chugging a large glass of it. Unfortunately, the only whittling going on wasn't around my waist, but around my tooth enamel.

Five months later . . .

As I stepped out of the shower I lifted the corner of my towel and wiped the foggy mirror. "Dammit, I'm still fat!" I groaned.

In that moment, I realized the solution was not going to be found on the cover of a tabloid magazine touting "Lose ten pounds in ten days," or any similar headline giving false hope.

Fortunately, my boyfriend cared enough to intervene. Mitch knew a secret . . . it's the same secret most competitive bodybuilders use to lose fat without sacrificing muscle mass.

He explained that strategic weekly doses of cake, cookies and ice cream were needed to correct my sluggish thyroid and improve my metabolism.

"Cake?!" I blurted. "Who doesn't like cake?"

I enthusiastically began a controlled dance between delayed gratification and carb-feeding frenzies.

My Transformation

Six months later and 20 pounds lighter, I was back at the doctor's office for my yearly checkup. Things were different. Every negative in my patient chart had been reversed. My blood work was optimal.

As she turned to leave the room, the doctor shook her head and smiled. "I don't know what you've been doing, but whatever it is, keep doing it."

Mischievously, I thought, "What I've been doing?

"I've been controlling carbs instead of carbs controlling me."

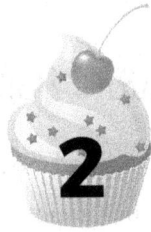

2

Laura's Story

My Lifelong Obsession with Donuts

Donuts are something you're supposed to grow out of, like eating lollipops the size of your head or ordering Sea Monkeys from the back of comic books.

After all, I am a 40-something-year-old woman. Aren't I supposed to have graduated to something more mature?

"It's not natural," I imagined the businesswoman in the pencil skirt hissing.

But I can't help it. To me, nothing compares to the humble donut and the joy it brings me.

Don't misunderstand. My relationship with donuts hasn't always been smooth sailing.

Over the years, several attempts have been made to keep us apart.

For starters, donuts and I never had my parents' full support. Donuts and other sugary delights were "the devil." It was a "gateway pastry," and if not thwarted, could lead to further sugary experimentation.

Jelly Donut - Beaufort, South Carolina, 1972

I was just five years old when I first met my soul mate.

I stood on my tippy toes as my tiny fingers gripped the cafeteria counter.

"Two jelly donuts, please," I chirped, my wispy blonde noggin and big blue eyes barely visible from the other side of the counter.

For some unexplainable reason, my private school served donuts to first-graders.

To be fair, it wasn't *all* first-graders. Most children ate what their parents told them to eat.

Not me; I craved jelly donuts and all their spastic side effects. Academic success, be damned!

Ever since I discovered the magic words "put it on my tab," an entire new world had opened up.

I had gone rogue.

Every morning I counted down the minutes until I could bust out of Mrs. Covington's reading class and hightail it across the large campus to the cafeteria.

I couldn't wait to eat those two soft jelly-filled donuts dusted lightly with powdered sugar. They made the rest of my ADHD-challenged day worth it.

Afraid that I wasn't heard the first time, I repeated my order slightly louder.

"Two jelly donuts, please."

Suddenly, the large lunch lady with the hair net leaned across the counter, her rubber index finger pointing down my button nose. "No more jelly donuts for you," she said in a stern voice.

"Wha- . . . what?" my mind reeled.

Apparently, my mom was curious why the same $1.25 charge posted on my account day after day, week after week. When she found out I was eating nothing but jelly donuts, she was furious.

"Your mother said, 'No more jelly donuts for you!'" she scolded.

It felt personal . . . like she had unknowingly risked her career by distributing contraband to prisoners.

The jelly donut gig was up.

Somehow, I'd have to find a way to get through the remainder of first grade without them.

Chocolate Cake Donut— Columbia, Missouri, 1976

Mom had secretly wished her grade school-aged daughters had possessed a talent she could actually be proud of.

Our mad playground tetherball skills weren't cutting it.

It was high time my older sister Barb and I began the transformation process from "ordinary" into graceful ballerinas or concert pianists.

Having previously crashed and burned in ballet, all bets were on piano.

If there was any silver lining to being forced to take piano lessons against my will, it was that they were located directly across the street from a Dunkin' Donuts.

For the next several weeks, I played along with my mom's charade, knowing that a chocolate cake donut was waiting at the end.

Between lessons, I found myself daydreaming about that magical chocolate cake covered in a blanket of thick chocolate icing.

Week after week, I ordered the same chocolate cake donut. Not because it was my favorite, but because I was too afraid to find out otherwise.

See, I wasn't sure how long my mom's piano prodigy experiment would last. And since piano lessons were my only connector to donuts, being adventurous wasn't a risk worth taking.

One wrong donut choice could be my last.

My weekly donut was the only sweet treat I was allowed to eat.

Dad had just finished paying off his medical school loans, and unnecessary dental bills for his four kids' cavities weren't part of the household budget. He believed just a whiff of sugar would cause his kids' teeth to instantly rot out of their heads.

Unfortunately, my parents were unified in their zero tolerance of sugar.

My mom's sugar hatred was so severe that it made the experience of ordering fast food an especially cringe-worthy ordeal.

"Would you like a Coke with your order?" the burger girl chirped.

You would have thought by my mom's reaction that the innocent teenager behind the counter was dealing cocaine to children.

"COKE?" she scolded. "Why, that's sugar water!" As if she didn't get it the first time and her kids weren't humiliated enough, she repeated, "Nothing but sugar water!"

So with the lure of donuts dangling like a sugar-infused carrot, I began bluffing my way through one piano lesson to the next.

"OK, Laura, let's hear the piece I gave you to practice," my teacher requested.

"One, two, three, four," I muttered. "One, two, three . . . "

"Stop counting your fingers," she said. "Start over, but this time without counting your fingers."

It was painfully obvious that no amount of piano lessons would move me closer to learning how to read sheet music.

"I don't think piano is really your thing," said my frazzled teacher. "Let's let this be your last lesson, OK?"

And with that, I was fired.

Fortunately, my sister turned out to be a pretty decent piano player. She actually practiced.

So thanks to Barb, my dream stayed alive for another ten chocolate cake donuts.

Chocolate Glazed Donut—Odessa, Texas, 1984

If there was any redeeming quality to Odessa, Texas, it was the Daylight Donuts shop next to the coin-op laundromat.

Odessa was never going to make it onto the pages of a lifestyle magazine. It was a combination of endless concrete and blowing sand.

But whatever Odessa lacked in culture, it more than made up for in football prowess.

My high school alma mater, Odessa Permian, was famous for collecting an insane number of Texas football state championships (1965, 1972, 1980, 1984, 1989, 1991). Hollywood even made a movie based on my beloved "Mojo" called *Friday Night Lights.*

Permian High School pep rallies were full-blown productions that rivaled some colleges'. The atmosphere, loud and frenzied, was like a raucous indoor Mardi Gras parade (sans the alcohol and beads).

There was only one thing that could pull me away from a Permian High School pep rally during my state championship-winning senior year . . . and that's donuts.

Fortunately, pep rallies created a unique one-hour window of opportunity to indulge my obsession. If I hurried, I could sneak out of the crowded, chaotic field house undetected.

Within 15 minutes, I could be across town and enjoying two or three of the most amazing chocolate glazed donuts I've ever eaten. They were so fresh they melted the second they touched my lips.

To most of the people I grew up with, not much justified living in Odessa beyond football championships. But to me, it will always be the donut shop next to the coin-op laundromat.

Plain Glazed Donut—Tulsa, Oklahoma, 1987

I was stuck. My new home was a college campus 600 miles away and I didn't have a car.

I was landlocked. Gone were the days when I could walk to the kitchen or drive to the nearest store for a snack.

Fortunately, my dorm housed a budding entrepreneur who could smell a good business opportunity.

Every Sunday, she would sit at the end of the hall in a folding chair selling plain glazed donuts.

Always stale. Always outrageously overpriced.

That didn't stop me from wanting to experience the euphoric feeling that's only possible from a rush of dopamine and crushing inflation.

Looking back, it was criminal what she charged. But I was desperate. I needed donuts at any cost, regardless of the quality.

My donut obsession rivaled a middle-aged woman's willingness to buy crappy tickets from a scalper to an Ed Sheeran concert.

At the end of the day, a bad donut is better than no donut at all.

Sprinkles Donut—Dallas, Texas, 2008

I did it for the money. That's why!

As a single mom of two grade school-aged boys, corporate America was able to provide something even more valuable than self-worth and a sense of purpose.

Why, Laura, what could be more valuable than purpose, you ask?

Easy: medical and dental benefits.

As anyone past 30 knows, maintenance becomes expensive. And unlike cars, our parts can't be traded in after accumulating a few thousand extra miles. Excluding cosmetic surgery, you get one set of factory parts and you need to make 'em last.

All kidding aside, corporate America provided something else equally valuable: donuts.

You thought I was going to say the "people," didn't you? Well, let me assure you, the people were just as important.

How else would we know when someone brought donuts to the office if not for that person? Every office has one.

"Donuts in the break room!" she'd yell. "Donuts in the break room!"

Under any other circumstance, that person would be nails-on-a-chalkboard-annoying. But on donut day, I wanted to hug her.

There's something particularly unique about a box of "corporate" donuts; they always contained loads of variety. It's as if they were subconsciously adhering to an unspoken anti-discrimination donut policy.

I imagined someone in HR saying, "Make sure you get at least one or two with nuts. We don't want problems."

I was drawn to the donuts with sprinkles. Just seeing them made me smile.

You see, in a buttoned-up corporate world that rewarded conformity, they were the artistic risk-takers who loved self-expression.

Like me, they hated red tape and longed for innovation and progress.

"I'd rather apologize than ask for permission," they'd say.

So, why did I, a creative person, spend well over a decade in corporate America, you ask?

I did it for the donuts. Sprinkle donuts.

Churros—McKinney, Texas, Present

For the past 15 years, I've been a minority among minorities.

My neighbors are mostly Mexican. I know "Mexican-American" is more PC, but I'm not sure that's accurate.

If you didn't experience my neighborhood firsthand, you'd swear it was cliché.

On any given day of the week, you could expect to see a Mexican man wearing a huge sombrero selling cinnamon-sugared churros from a pushcart.

Tejano music blared so loudly you'd swear it was Oktoberfest. Apparently, Germans and Mexicans have something in common: They both love the accordion.

It's true, I live in a loud and often chaotic place, but my neighbors are without pretense, which I absolutely love.

Trust me, nobody is trying hard to "Keep up with the Hernandezes."

Best of all are the perks. Besides the obvious absence of HOA fees, it's located a block from my favorite donut shop. Best Donuts was a business that actually lives up to its name.

For over a decade, the same Chinese lady has greeted me at the counter with her signature brown apron and broad smile.

"What donut you want?" she'd ask.

Fearing the fat-gaining repercussions of eating them myself, I'd mostly buy for my two young sons. (Yep, I passed along my donut-loving gene.)

I had convinced myself that I was content with experiencing donuts through my other senses, sans my taste buds.

"Mmmmmmm!" I'd say, inhaling deeply. "I can almost taste them!"

That was until I discovered the Carb Party Diet.

Now, every Friday night my last thought before I drift off to sleep is, "When I wake up, I'm killing me some donuts!"

And maybe later, if the Mexican man in the sombrero is around, a churro, too!

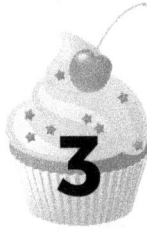

3

. . . .

Why Diets Fail

Here's why most diets fail: They practically require you be married to a low-carb lifestyle and vow to never eat carbs again!

"I, (*your name*), promise to love, honor and cherish Meat and Green Leafy Vegetables until death do us part."

Gone are your commitment-free days carelessly enjoying guilt-free chips and margaritas on Friday nights with your girlfriends.

Nope, you're married now, and for the sake of your marriage, concessions need to be made.

Remember, you vowed: "Until death do us part."

"Besides," you reason, "I'm in love!" Matter of fact, you're downright giddy. Just the thought of losing 15 pounds of fat makes your heart skip a beat.

With your fist raised high, you scream, "Dammit if I'll be a diet statistic!"

And then it happens: Just a few days into your new diet, you *cheat!*

The dozen warm, gooey donuts in your office break room prove too much of a temptation. "I'm only human!" you justify.

Soon you find you're headlong into a passionate affair with carbs.

You sit behind your office desk fantasizing about your next cookie "quickie." Every night you sneak out of bed for a tryst in your kitchen pantry. Soon your cheating heart is on full display while you make out with a quart of Rocky Road ice cream in full view of your husband and kids.

The roller-coaster surge of blood sugar causes your hunger hormone ghrelin (which acts like a gremlin) to spike, sending your cravings spiraling out of control.

Your brain starts yelling, "I'm starving," and you literally feel your very survival depends on how quickly you can get to the nearest fast-food drive-thru.

Within days, you wind up gaining back all the weight you lost plus some.

"But I'm different," you plead. "I'm no cheater!"

OK. So let's say you don't have a wandering eye. You stayed faithful to your low-carb vows.

That's admirable, commendable, and a host of other complimentary words.

But guess what? Your low-carb diet is still destined to fail.

You see, even if *you* don't cheat, your thyroid gland will cheat on you.

As a result of your long-term, steadfast commitment to banish carbs and your monogamous relationship with meat, your fat-burning hormones begin to reverse. Your thyroid produces less and less leptin (your main fat-burning hormone), which signals your body to pack on more fat.

Good news! None of the above has to happen.

The Carb Party Diet's secret weapon is *carbs!*

It stokes the flames of your fat-burning hormones by revealing the precise time to strategically "fall off the low-carb wagon" and into a sinfully delicious dessert tray to keep your thyroid healthy and leptin levels high.

By eating carbs with intention, at exactly the perfect time, your fat melts away easier and gaining fat becomes much more difficult.

The cake is still there and, yes, you can eat it too!

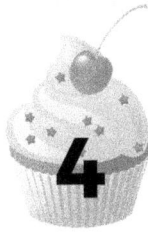

. . . .

The Fat Truth about Leptin

Recently, there's been a lot of buzz about leptin, considered the master fat-loss hormone. In fact, just including the word "leptin" on a book cover has made millions of dollars. It's marketing fairy dust!

Meanwhile, insulin, an equally important fat-burning hormone has been kicked to the curb.

I guess, in terms of marketing hype, it's "so last decade." It's as if the diet industry is going through a mid-life crisis and wants to be seen with a sexier, more head-turning piece of arm candy—and her name is leptin.

Truth is, insulin and leptin are a power couple. They're inseparable and their powers can be used for good or evil.

For instance, Brad Pitt and Angelina Jolie, a celebrity power couple, use their powers for good by providing humanitarian aid around the world. On the other hand, outlaws Bonnie &

Clyde used their powers for evil, causing nothing but death and destruction.

You see, it's impossible to talk about one fat-burning hormone without talking about the other. They're both important independent of each other.

Unfortunately, most overweight people have screwed up both hormones and subsequently hijacked their weight-loss efforts.

Years of eating a high-carbohydrate diet have led to a condition called insulin resistance, a condition in which the pancreas produces insulin but the body doesn't respond to it properly. In some extreme cases it can lead to type 2 diabetes and require insulin shots.

Like fat-burning dominos, insulin resistance is correlated to a phenomenon called leptin resistance, in which your fat makes plenty of leptin but your brain doesn't see it.

As a result of perceived low leptin levels, your brain thinks you're starving. You can never eat enough to match your uncontrollable hunger. The more you eat, the fatter you get, and the fatter you get—the higher your leptin levels soar. It's a vicious cycle that, if left unchecked, will eventually lead to obesity.

Resetting Your Metabolism

So what's the answer? How do you overhaul your hormones?

Simple: Keep your insulin down. And the best way to keep insulin levels down is by not allowing them to go up. Insulin arrives on the scene the second your blood sugar level rises. In other words—stop eating sugar! (Or carbs that convert to sugar.)

But WAIT, won't six consecutive days of ultra-low carbs make leptin levels plummet? And if leptin levels are low, won't fat loss become more difficult?

Yep, that's exactly right.

That's why you *need* a Carb Party. Each strategic carb re-feed is like hitting a big red reset button to restore your leptin to normal levels. Your perfectly timed Carb Party stokes the flames of your fat-burning furnace and keeps your hormones functioning at optimal levels. So start planning out all the chocolaty, decadent, sweet treats that you'll eat in seven days. Your fat-burning hormones will thank you for it!

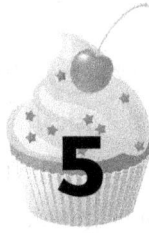

5

• • • •

Eat Cake, Lose Weight

I still remember how my best friend Natasha just stood there staring at me, her mouth wide open.

"Hold up, Hannah. Let me get this straight," she said. "You're now a size-four-skinny *because* you eat cookies, cake, and ice cream?"

I smiled and nodded. "Every Saturday night! It's like hitting a big, red, reset button on my metabolism. I'm a 24/7 fat-burning machine."

I raised my T-shirt to expose my abs. "My weekly 'binge-fest' does this . . . without sit-ups, Zumba or crazy cardio!"

She could hardly believe what she was hearing and seeing. She had just endured a diet that required her to give up all her favorite foods for a whole 30 days.

And here I was, lean, toned, and full of energy.

Excited, I explained, "Every seventh night I eat things like fresh baked bread, fruit, rice, pizza, snickerdoodle cookies,

Rice Krispies treats, gummy bears, chocolate, cinnamon rolls, donuts, and french fries . . . basically anything I crave."

Natasha was at her wits' end. She remembered how hard it was white-knuckling through each 24 hours without carbohydrates—which made her b*itchy and miserable all day—just to gain the weight back plus ten pounds.

Truthfully, I could sympathize with her skepticism. I remember thinking, "Oh, great, another fad diet." I had tried and failed every diet at least once. Believe me, I know—my struggle started when I was 14.

Even after swearing off bread and dessert, and exercising for hours each week, I could never lose the muffin top that spilled over the waistband of my favorite jeans.

I didn't know the secret was *carbs*, specifically when to have my next intentional wheels-off Carb Party.

Now I enjoy all my favorite foods including cookies, cake and ice cream, and have never been skinnier, healthier and stronger!

Consider this your personal invitation to join my next Carb Party. I guarantee you'll not only lose fat, but you'll have a ton of fun.

You can literally party your a** off!

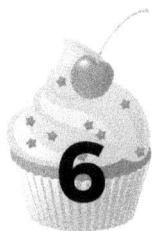

6

. . . .

If Dr. Atkins &
Little Debbie Had a Baby . . .

Hannah: Don't you wish diets could be explained like a Hollywood movie logline?

Laura: You mean something like this (cue movie soundtrack): "The Carb Party Diet, a tale of two ordinary women who take an epic seven-day fat-burning journey . . . a journey which will require traversing a series of obstacles and challenges such as resisting a delicious pastry platter of muffins, scones, and cinnamon rolls during a soul-sucking Monday morning conference call, or resisting the temptation to devour an entire box of chocolate chip cookies for getting the baby to finally fall asleep after two hours of singing the same lullaby like a broken record. Ultimately it's a 'feel-good-chick-flick-buddy-comedy' with a happy ending. During the seventh day of the journey, our heroes finally arrive at their destination and enjoy an over-the-top Carb Party; bingeing on brownies, cookies, cupcakes, muffins, ice cream, chocolate, and wine." (Be sure to watch the credits at the end—Hannah and Laura's carb drunk outtakes are hilarious!)

Hannah: Or perhaps you could simply use this logline: "Dr. Atkins meets Little Debbie"? Boom, there it is!

Days 1-9: Induction

During the first 9½ days, your *main focus* should be about eating an ultra-low-carbohydrate diet to deplete glucose, your body's primary fuel source. Eat no more than 20 grams of carbs per day.

During this phase, you're programming your body to burn dietary fat and stored body fat as fuel, a process known as fat adaptation. If you eat carbs during the induction phase, you'll raise your insulin, which will bring the fat-burning process to a screeching halt. Don't do it. You deserve the great results that delayed gratification will provide.

Next, choose which day of the week you want to have your first Carb Party. This is the day you'll "carb out" and eat all your favorite foods. As a result of eating carbs you'll spike your insulin and keep your fat-burning hormones healthy.

Laura: I chose Saturday as my Carb Party day because it's convenient. I like to let loose with my friends and the weekends are the only time that works.

Hannah: Yeah, Saturdays always made the most sense. Who wants to be doing Carb Party by yourself on Monday behind an office desk?

Ultimately, your protein and fat grams should typically be at a 1:1 ratio. This means your diet should mostly consist of equal amounts of fat and protein. In other words, restrict your meals and snacks to only meat, oil, and fatty cheeses.

APPROVED VEGGIES: Asparagus, avocado, green bell pepper, broccoli, cabbage, celery, collard greens, cauliflower, cucumber, kale, lettuce, mushrooms, onion, sauerkraut, spaghetti squash, spinach, tomato, yellow squash, and zucchini.

AVOID: Fruit, sugar, honey, starchy vegetables, meal replacement shakes, bread, meal replacement bars, protein bars, half-and-half, coconut milk, almond milk, milk . . . anything with the word "milk."

IMPORTANT: During this induction phase, restrict your carbs to 20 grams or fewer per day. If in doubt, always check the nutrition label for the total number of carbohydrate grams.

Hannah: If you're like most women, you're asking, "OMG, if I can't eat carbs, what can I eat?"

Laura: Easy. Basically anything with a heartbeat.

Hannah: I think what you're trying to say is you can eat anything that *previously* had a heartbeat.

Laura: Good point, I don't think anyone wants their steak that fresh!

Hannah: Yeah, otherwise it would moo.

Laura: While we're talking meat, I know most women wonder if it's possible to eat *too* much meat.

Hannah: I always say, let your inner carnivore be your guide.

Laura: Yeah, but you're definitely not a "normal" carnivore . . .

Hannah: I know, I'm part T-Rex! I can eat a pound of beef, no problem. But you're right, most women are afraid that if they eat that much meat they'll be eating too much fat. Their fear is that fat will make them fat. You know, like that saying we all grew up with: "You are what you eat."

Laura: Yikes, if that were true, I'd be a donut.

Hannah: And I'd be a cow.

Laura: Moo! All kidding aside, eating fat doesn't make you fat. It's actually a good thing. First of all, fat has zero impact on insulin. And, fat is extremely satiating. It's nearly impossible to binge-eat on fat alone.

Hannah: Right. When was the last time you sat on the couch with a large tub of butter and a spoon?

Day 10: Carb Party Beginning at 5:00 p.m.

Carb Party [kahrb] [pahr-tee]
   Noun: a social gathering scheduled every seven days with your friends and/or family for the sole purpose of eating unlimited quantities of carbohydrates.

Starting no earlier than 5:00 p.m., you may begin eating all your favorite carbs, including but not limited to: BBQ baked beans, pancakes, fruit juice, cupcakes, waffles, Popsicles, chocolate, wine, chips & salsa, beer, soda, sherbet, potato chips, cookies, margaritas, rice, fresh fruit, cereal, tortillas, tacos, oatmeal, funnel cake, fresh baked bread, banana nut muffins, pretzels, ice cream, peanut butter, pasta, popcorn, brownies, pizza, s'mores, crackers, apple pie, baklava, flan, yogurt parfaits, granola, candy, churros, or anything else your little carb-starved heart desires.

Carb Drunk [karb] [druhngk]

Adjective: a temporary state of mental and physical impairment caused by eating carbs after an extended period of carb sobriety.

Example: Jude was so carb drunk that we saw her passed out in the corner of the media room with chocolate smeared all over her face.

Noun: a carb-loaded person.

Example: Every Carb Party has at least one Carb Drunk.

Laura: I think I know why we usually stay home and do a Mix & Match Carb Party (see Chapter 13, "52 Carb Party Ideas").

Hannah: Why's that?

Laura: Because we're always carb drunk within the first 30 minutes of the Carb Party . . .

Hannah: I know, right? The house always looks like a CSI crime scene—the kitchen ransacked and bodies are sprawled out all over the floor.

Laura: You'd think we were all shot with elephant tranquilizer darts!

Hannah: Or chipmunk darts since we're all smaller now!

Days 11-16: Low Carb

Restrict yourself to no more than 30 grams of carbs per day for the next six consecutive days.

Again, the main objective is to keep your blood sugar levels consistently low. Eating carbs will trigger your body to release insulin, which signals the fat storage process.

Hannah: Hey, Laura, do you remember my 'carboholic' friend?

Laura: Which one? The one who carries "emergency chocolate" in her purse?

Hannah: Yep, that's the one. She practically had a panic attack when I said I eat low-carb during my workweek.

Laura: Did you have to revive her with chocolate?

Hannah: Almost, but then I explained that she could do anything for six days.

Laura: (sarcasm) I can think of a few things that we endure for six days that are slightly (sarcasm) more painful.

Hannah: (sarcasm) Umm, like maybe your period?

Laura: (sarcasm) Yeah, and we get to enjoy that for a solid week, every month, for years . . .

Hannah: (sarcasm) Woo hoo!

Day 17: Carb Party Time!

Again, beginning no earlier than 5:00 p.m., enjoy all your favorite starchy-sweet treats you've been dreaming about for a week.

Laura: Remember celebrating Natasha's birthday during Carb Party?

Hannah: That girl sure loves her fruity cocktails!

Laura: We made her wear that message-T: "Designated Drinker!"

Hannah: Yeah, but after her third frozen margarita—was it really necessary?

Laura: *Thank goodness for Uber!*

NOTE: If you need party theme inspiration, refer to Chapter 13, "52 Carb Party Ideas."

Rinse and Repeat

Follow a 6:1 protocol for as long as needed or desired. This means six days of eating mostly fat and protein foods. You should consume no more than 30 carbohydrates per day followed by one noncontinuous Carb Party beginning no earlier than 5:00 p.m.

In summary, strip the carbs out of your diet for six days to keep your insulin consistently low, followed with a weekly Carb Party on day seven. Continue the above process as few or as many times as you desire.

We understand that life happens. So, even if vacations or other planned or unplanned occasions interrupt your weekly Carb Parties, don't stress out. You can always use the Carb Party Diet as a tool to get you back on track.

Fat-Torching Tip: For even better fat-burning results, restrict your Carb Party treats to foods that are *nonfat* (i.e., fruit, mashed potatoes, baked potatoes, rice, pasta, bread, gummy bears, hard candy, taffy, lollipops, Popsicles, fruity cocktails, frozen adult beverages, sorbet, or sherbet) and avoid high-fat, high-carb options like ice cream, french fries, or homemade fudge. To be clear, you can enjoy *any* carb treat you like and the Carb Party Diet will keep your metabolism revved up, but for even faster fat loss, opt for low-fat carbolicious treats.

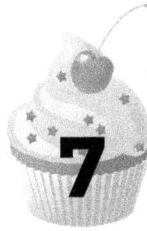

7

· · · ·

How to "Carb Party Diet"
(. . . and Lose Your Muffin Top!)

Days 1-10

Induction Phase - 10 Days

During days 1-10 you will follow a 9 & 1 protocol. This means nine days of carb depletion (20 carb grams or less) followed by a Carb Party, a carbohydrate re-feed day beginning no earlier than 5:00 p.m.

You can choose any low-carb, high-fat/protein foods to eat during your nine carb-stripping days. The purpose of abstaining from carbohydrates is to make your body more fat-adaptive (efficient at burning fat). I've provided a sample menu if you'd like to see what Hannah or I would eat on any given week. Again, continue eating fewer than 20 carbohydrates daily for nine consecutive days.

On your designated Carb Party day you can eat however you would normally eat PLUS anything carbolicious (containing carbs) that you've been craving during the previous nine low-carb days. Refer to Chapter 13, "52 Carb Party Ideas," if you would like to "Carb Party" with friends or family. The purpose of this carb re-feed is to cause a dramatic spike in insulin. Strategic carb re-feeds keep your thyroid healthy. A healthy thyroid is necessary to keep your leptin levels optimal for greater fat burning potential.

Weeks 1-4

Weeks 1-4: 6 & 1 Protocol – 1:1 Fat/Protein

During weeks 1-4 you will follow a 6 & 1 protocol. This means six consecutive days of low-carb (30 grams or less) eating followed by one day of high-carbohydrate consumption beginning no earlier than 5:00 p.m.

You can choose any combination of protein and fats to eat during your deficit days as well as on your Carb Party. Aim for a 1:1 ratio of fat to protein and no more than 30 carbs per day. (See approved vegetable list.) The purpose of abstaining from carbohydrates is to make your body more fat-adaptive (efficient at burning fat). I've also provided a sample meal plan as an example of a structured guess-free meal schedule.

On your designated Carb Party you can eat however you would normally eat *plus* anything carbolicious (containing carbs) that you've been craving during the previous six low-carb days. Refer to Chapter 13, "52 Carb Party ideas," if you would like to do group Carb Parties. The purpose of this carb re-feed is to cause a dramatic spike in insulin which will keep your thyroid healthy. A healthy thyroid will keep your leptin at peak levels so your body can burn more fat during the following four to six days.

Skip breakfast: Delaying your first meal forces your body to start burning more body fat and improves your leptin sensitivity. Fat loss becomes easier and fat storage more difficult.

Weeks 5-7

Weeks 5-7: 6 & 1 Carb Protocol – 2:1 Fat/Protein

During weeks 5 through 7, you will continue to follow a 6 & 1 protocol. This means six days of avoiding dietary carbohydrates (30 grams or less) followed with one nonconsecutive day where you are aiming to eat higher carbohydrates beginning at 5:00 p.m.

Aim for a 2:1 ratio of fat to protein. This is easier said than done. Most people aren't used to eating excessive amounts of fat. When that fat is combined with carbohydrates (e.g., mashed potatoes with butter, french fries, ice cream or cookies), weight-loss progress can stall.

The best way to get more dietary fat is to choose heavy whipping cream in your coffee, cook in bacon or coconut oil, and choose fattier cuts of beef or pork.

Again, weekends work best for most people to enjoy your Carb Party, as this is when most people like to relax and be entertained. Choosing a non-workday will also be more convenient for doing a Carb Party with a supportive group of friends, co-workers, and family members.

For example: Saturday or Sunday as opposed to Monday, Tuesday, Wednesday, Thursday, or Friday . . .

Weeks 8-9

Weeks 8-9: 6 & 1 Protocol – 1:1 Fat/Protein

During weeks 8 and 9 you will follow a 6 & 1 protocol. This means six days of low-carb eating plus one day of high-carb eating beginning no earlier than 5:00 p.m.

You can choose any foods to eat during your deficit days as long as they don't exceed 30 grams of carbs per day. Refer to the one-week sample meal plan if you want guidance on how to plan your six low-carb days.

Read food labels to find the total number of carbs contained. Avoid packaged and processed foods, which are notorious for containing an excess of blatant and hidden carbs.

On the day of your Carb Party—enjoy all the carbs you've been craving during the previous six days, beginning at 5:00 p.m. Refer to Chapter 13, "52 Carb Party Ideas," if you need party theme ideas to celebrate with your friends and family.

Weeks 10-12

Weeks 10-12: 6 & 1 Protocol – 1:1 Fat/Protein

Congratulations!! I bet you are looking and feeling so much better now that you have reduced your total sugar over the course of almost three months. Way to go!!!

During weeks 10 through 12 you will continue following a 6 & 1 protocol. This means six days of ultra-low-carb eating followed by one non-consecutive high carbohydrate day beginning no earlier than 5:00 p.m. Strive for a 1:1 ratio of fat to protein and no more than 30 carbs per day.

CARB PARTY FAT-TORCHING TIP: Choose lower fat treats during your Carb Party such as: fruit, mashed potatoes, baked potatoes, dried fruit, Popsicles, gelato, low-fat yogurt, pasta, rice, and movie theater-type candy.

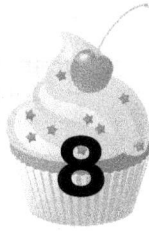

8

• • • •

The Lazy Dieter's Way
to Lose Belly Fat

Think of the following chart as a sort of flab-busting roadmap to navigate your way through a 12-week Carb Party Diet journey. During the first "official week" (following induction phase) of your **buddy road trip,** limit your food choices to primarily proteins and fat-like meats, cheeses, and oils (i.e., grilled chicken, bun-less burgers, turkey lettuce wraps, pork chops, salmon fillet, grilled trout, baked cod, grilled shrimp, avocados, bacon, and mozzarella sticks). On the seventh day, get together with your girlfriends or family members and celebrate with a Carb Party! No earlier than 5:00 p.m., begin enjoying your carb favorites that you delayed eating during the previous six days. Get creative! Choose any one of the 52 Carb Party Ideas provided in Chapter 13 or combine them all to boost your leptin levels and keep your thyroid happy and healthy for weeks to come.

Losing weight has never been so carbolicious!

Week	Mon-Fri	Saturday	Sunday
1	Protein/Fat	CARBS	Protein/Fat
2	Protein/Fat	CARBS	Protein/Fat
3	Protein/Fat	CARBS	Protein/Fat
4	Protein/Fat	CARBS	Protein/Fat
5	Fat/Protein	CARBS	Protein/Fat
6	Fat/Protein	CARBS	Protein/Fat
7	Fat/Protein	CARBS	Protein/Fat
8	Protein/Fat	CARBS	Protein/Fat
9	Protein/Fat	CARBS	Protein/Fat
10	Protein/Fat	CARBS	Protein/Fat
11	Protein/Fat	CARBS	Protein/Fat
12	Protein/Fat	CARBS	Protein/Fat

Fat-Torching Tip

Skip breakfast: Delay your first meal to force your body to start burning more body fat and improve your leptin sensitivity. Fat loss will become easier and fat storage more difficult.

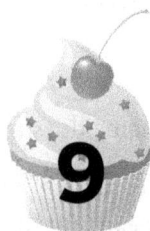

9

• • • •

Three Shortcuts to Weight-Loss Success

"An ounce of prevention is worth a pound of cure."

–Ben Franklin

Weight-loss temptations are everywhere: your car's cup holder, the office break room, restaurant menus, and in the aisles of your favorite grocery store. The last place you should be tempted is in your own home. It should be your personal weight-loss sanctuary. To ensure your home is "Carb Party-friendly," heed Ben's advice: apply "an ounce of prevention" and watch the excess pounds disappear.

Organizing

FRIDGE & PANTRY: Remember playing hide-n-seek when you were a kid? That's what you're going to play with all your carby foods like chips, cookies, candy, crackers, cereal, fruit snacks, rice, pasta, syrup, and sauces. However, unlike the game of your youth, this game doesn't end when it starts to get dark; it lasts all week long. Start by separating all those tasty carb temptations that you can't eat during the majority of your week and place them somewhere else. The idea is "out of sight, out of mind." Either store them on a high pantry shelf or place them in a plastic storage bin labeled 'Carb Party.' Don't worry, these items aren't going MIA; they'll come out and play with you again on the evening of your Carb Party.

SPICE RACK: Your diet will consist predominantly of protein and fat, so you'll want to have tasty seasonings to keep things interesting.

Identify your top five favorite flavors to spice up chicken, beef, pork and fish. These spices will need to be within arm's reach as your "go-to" seasonings.

Some recommended spices: garlic powder, red pepper powder, black pepper, any meat rub WITHOUT sugar, and salt. Tabasco, Frank's RedHot, or Sriracha sauce. Our favorite all-purpose gluten-free, sugar-free, carb-free meat rub/seasoning is Spain's Smokehouse Original Seasoning.

Shopping

Create a weekly shopping list of low-carb foods. These items are typically whole foods such as eggs, bacon, chicken, beef, fish, cheese, butter, coffee, and heavy whipping cream. You'll want to buy enough of each item to last a week. We suggest you buy in bulk to save time and money.

Sample Shopping List

Sam's Club or Costco

- Chicken breast
- Sausage
- Steak
- Ground beef
- Chicken broth
- Canned chicken breast
- Mayo
- Mustard
- Shredded cheese
- Cheese sticks or slices
- Frozen cod
- Frozen salmon
- Frozen sea bass
- Bacon
- Eggs
- Avocados
- Frozen broccoli
- Fresh spinach
- Fresh coleslaw
- Sour cream
- Heavy whipping cream
- Coconut oil
- Olive oil
- Spring water
- Spices

*CP Tip: Check out online farm-to-table delivery services like FreshDirect, which will deliver meat and vegetables to your doorstep and avoid busy checkout lines and crowded parking lots (limited availability).

*CP Tip: Identify foods that your entire household would enjoy regardless of whether they're doing a Carb Party (e.g., grilled chicken prepared with olive oil and Italian seasoning).

*CP Tip: Bring your shopping list with you.

*CP Tip: Shop on the outer edges of the store (i.e., produce, meats, and dairy) to avoid high-carb prepackaged foods.

*CP Tip: Shop on a full stomach to avoid impulse buys.

Prepping

As the saying goes, "If you fail to plan, you plan to fail."

Failing to prep low-carb meals in advance, you will end up grabbing whatever convenient, sugar-laden, carb-dense item is within reach.

Spontaneity is great if you're an improv (improvisational) actor, but not so great for every other area of life.

Think about it. Which are you more likely to spontaneously to eat: the convenient box of cookies sitting in your pantry or the low-carbohydrate meal that hasn't yet been prepared?

So, how exactly can you avoid "falling off the wagon" and into a plate of pasta?

Simple: Plan your weekly meals ahead of time.

By planning and preparing your meals in bulk, you are essentially making homemade low-carb frozen meals. As a result, you will be less likely to give in to the temptation to splurge on high-carb foods during the week, and save loads of time and money in the process.

Here's how: Cook three to six days' worth of meals either on a Sunday afternoon and/or on Wednesday night. The option to prep twice per week would allow you variety and flexibility. By cooking only three meals at a time, you can eat out for business or social reasons without wasting food.

Next: Break down a bulk meal into individual portions for lunches and dinners. This means you'll need a minimum of six containers to make three lunches and three dinners for the week. Make sure your refrigerator is organized so your meals are clearly visible. Seeing your low-carb meals motivates you to stay on track, in the same way that visible high-carb treats are a diet-wrecking temptation.

*CP Tip: Invest in a cast-iron skillet to add more flavor to meats.

*CP Tip: Save bacon grease for cooking chicken & beef.

*CP Tip: Cook with an induction stove top to speed cooking time.

*CP Bonus Tip: Take a "before" Carb Party Diet photo wearing a swimsuit and hide the scale. Scales don't specify what is being measured (i.e., fat, water, or muscle).

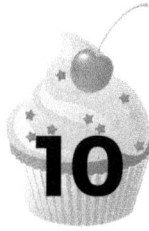

10

. . . .

One Week Sample Menu

Unlike all the other diet books and programs before this one, we don't believe in force-feeding (pun intended) women a rigid and controlling diet. We believe in *empowering* women with the right information and tools so they can make their own decisions. It's your body, not ours, after all!

With that said, the following is merely a seven-day sample menu:

SUNDAY - Rest [-aurant] Day

BREAKFAST

- Starbucks – Tall Americano

LUNCH

- Chipotle – Bowl (without rice, beans or flour/corn tortilla)
- Double chicken, sour cream, red hot sauce, guacamole, lettuce, cheese, grilled fajita peppers & onions
- One multivitamin

DINNER

- In-N-Out Burger – Double Protein Style Burger (without bun), no fries!!

Laura: I personally hate to cook so I'm eating fast food quite a bit during the week. Since I'm usually in the drive-thru, the easiest way to order a low-carb burger (or sandwich) is to say, "Hamburger, no bun, extra lettuce, please."

MONDAY

BREAKFAST

- Scrambled eggs
- Two slices of bacon
- Coffee with heavy whipping cream
- One multivitamin

LUNCH

- Grilled smoked sausage with mustard

DINNER

- Frozen cod with butter, salt, pepper

TUESDAY

BREAKFAST

- Fried eggs
- Coffee, black

LUNCH

- Four slices of bacon
- Avocado seasoned with red pepper, salt, pepper
- One multivitamin

DINNER

- Rotisserie chicken
- Steamed spinach with butter

Laura: You started your day with eggs and ended it with rotisserie chicken. OMG, that's cradle-to-grave dining!

Hannah: Circle of life!

Laura: Hakuna matata!

WEDNESDAY

BREAKFAST

- Coffee – Splenda, heavy whipping cream
- Two eggs

LUNCH

- Homemade chicken salad (no bread)
- One multivitamin

DINNER

- Grilled salmon, broccoli with butter

THURSDAY

BREAKFAST

- Cold-brewed coffee – Splenda, heavy whipping cream
- Loaded eggs with breakfast sausage

LUNCH

- Avocado seasoned with red pepper, salt, black pepper
- One-half pound of beef, seasoned to taste
- One multivitamin

DINNER

- One frozen sea bass fillet seasoned with salt, pepper, and extra butter

Laura: Sea bass? What a fish snob!

Hannah: Well, as long as this is a *sample menu*, I may as well dream big!

FRIDAY

BREAKFAST

- Sugar-free flavored "coffee of the day" with heavy whipping cream

LUNCH

- Four slices of bacon
- Two scrambled eggs seasoned with red pepper, salt, black pepper, and a little leftover bacon grease
- One multivitamin

DINNER

- Frozen blackened salmon fillet topped with cream cheese and avocado

Hannah: OK, who's the fish snob now?

Laura: Relax! It's frozen and I buy mine at Sam's Club.

SATURDAY - CARB PARTY DAY

BREAKFAST

- Double-shot espresso Tall Americano

LUNCH

- Grilled chicken salad
- One multivitamin

Hannah: Just a friendly warning: watch out for those sneaky restaurant salads loaded with croutons or tortilla strips. And always ask for low-carb salad dressing. Or to be on the safe side, request a side of vinegar and oil.

5:00 p.m. CARB PARTY

#8 "Breakfast for Dinner Party"

- Peanut butter chocolate chip banana muffins, pancakes, strawberry waffles, Nutella banana waffles, French toast with maple syrup & powdered sugar, chocolate cake donuts, and cinnamon rolls.

Hannah: I'm glad I skipped breakfast this morning!

Laura: I know, me too! I'm really looking forward to *donuts*!

Hannah: Calm down, Homer!

Laura: "Hmm . . . jelly donuts!"

What are you gonna eat? Let me rephrase that—what are you going to eat besides peanut butter chocolate chip banana muffins?

Hannah: OK, how about a ginormous stack of homemade chocolate chip waffles topped with a side of Nutella and sliced bananas. And oh, I almost forgot; they need to be swimming in syrup.

Laura: I'm glad we decided to do the Breakfast for Dinner Party; PJs have elastic waistbands!

Sample Menu Chart

Some people are more visual than others and appreciate seeing the same information in charts or graphs. If this is you, substitute the above menu with this handy chart.

Day	Breakfast	Lunch	Dinner
Sun	• Coffee, black, or heavy whipping cream	• Chipotle Bowl (any meat desired) fajita • Cheese, sour cream, lettuce, salsa, guacamole • Multivitamin	• In-N-Out Burger, Double Meat Protein Style Burger (no bun)
Mon	• 2 Scrambled eggs & 1 slice of bacon • Coffee with heavy whipping cream	• Grilled smoked sausage with mustard • Broccoli with butter • Multivitamin	• Frozen cod seasoned with lemon pepper, butter, and salt • Cauliflower
Tue	• Coffee, black, or heavy whipping cream • 2 Fried eggs	• 4 Slices of bacon • Avocado with salt and pepper • Multivitamin	• Rotisserie chicken • 1 Cup steamed spinach with butter
Wed	• Coffee – Splenda, heavy whipping cream	• 2 Eggs – any style • 4 Slices of bacon • Multivitamin	• Homemade chicken salad on a bed of lettuce

Day	Breakfast	Lunch	Dinner
Thu	• Cold-brewed coffee – Splenda, heavy whipping cream • Loaded eggs with breakfast sausage	• Avocado seasoned with red pepper, salt, black pepper • ½ Lb. beef, seasoned to taste • Multivitamin	• 1 Frozen sea bass fillet seasoned with salt, pepper, and extra butter • Steamed spinach with butter, salt and pepper
Fri	• Sugar-free flavored "coffee of the day" with heavy whipping cream	• 2 Scrambled eggs seasoned with red pepper, salt, and black pepper, and a little leftover bacon grease • Multivitamin	• Frozen blackened salmon fillet topped with cream cheese and small avocado
Sat	• Coffee, • 2 Scrambled eggs	**CARB PARTY 5:00 p.m.** • Peanut butter chocolate chip banana muffins, pancakes, strawberry waffles	• Nutella banana waffles, • French toast with maple syrup & powdered sugar, chocolate cake donuts, and cinnamon rolls

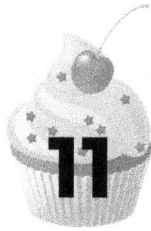

. . . .

11

Low-Carb Restaurant Survival Guide

At some point between Carb Parties you're going to find yourself at a restaurant. Don't panic! There are plenty of low-carb entrees you can eat; you just need to know how to recognize them. For instance, almost every popular chain restaurant or locally owned café utilizes meat and vegetables for their menu items. The trick is to identify meaty entrees first and then pair them with Carb Party-friendly vegetables.

Using the following guidelines, you too can safely navigate your way through any fast-food drive-thru or five star restaurant menu:

Breakfast = Meat + Vegetables + Fat

Meat: eggs (any style), omelet, frittata, bacon, sausage, ham, chicken, beef, pork, fish

Vegetables: asparagus, avocado, green bell pepper, broccoli, cabbage, celery, collard greens, cauliflower, cucumber, kale, lettuce, mushrooms, onion, sauerkraut, spaghetti squash, spinach, tomato, yellow squash, zucchini

Fat: cheese, butter, olive oil, coconut oil, mayo

Lunch/Dinner = Meat + Vegetables + Fat

Meat: Beef, pork, chicken, seafood, fajitas, tuna salad, grilled tuna, pork chops, meatloaf, grilled steak, meatballs, sausage, salads, burgers & sandwiches (no bun!)

Vegetables: Asparagus, avocado, green bell pepper, broccoli, cabbage, celery, collard greens, cauliflower, cucumber, kale, lettuce, mushrooms, onion, sauerkraut, spaghetti squash, spinach, tomato, yellow squash, zucchini

Fat: Butter, olive oil, coconut oil, mayo

Avoid These Menu Items

Baked bread, beans, burger buns, biscuits, sugar-coated nuts, corn, crackers, chips, croutons, fruit, pasta, pitas, potatoes, rice, toast, tortillas, juice, wine, cocktails, soda, and sweet tea. (Avoid any breaded meats!)

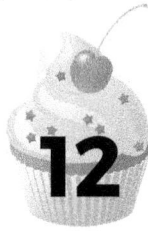

12

• • • •

Dear Carb Party Diary

(DAY 49) Tonight I wanted to record everything that happened leading up to this week's Carb Party. My fear is, if I don't write it all down before I fall asleep, I might forget. I hope this all makes sense later when I'm "sugar sober." I won't lie—I'm pretty Carb Drunk! Here goes . . .

T-minus five hours to Carb Party

This morning I rubbed the sleep from my eyes, grabbed my Carb Party wish list from off the nightstand and stumbled to the kitchen. I stood barefoot and began checking my Carb Party inventory: "Gummy Bears, check!" "Rice Krispies treats, check!" "Chocolate, check!" "Wine, check!"

Next, I looked in the refrigerator. "Slice 'n bake cookies, check. Milk, check!"

Then I scanned the freezer. "Sea salt caramel gelato, check! Gluten-free ice cream sandwiches, check."

I wrote a quick note on the bottom of the list: "Don't forget to bring the rice cooker and to run through the drive-thru for french fries."

I marked my "maybe" items with a yellow highlighter: Pizza, cinnamon-swirled raisin toast, chocolate donuts and banana nut muffins.

Throughout the afternoon, my Carb Party friends began bombarding my phone with "food porn" pictures. Why do we always insist on torturing each other like this?

I scrolled through endless pictures of fresh-baked brownies, bottles of wine, ice cream sundaes, cupcakes, cinnamon rolls, gourmet donuts, DIY s'mores dip, overflowing bowls of candy, and chocolate-covered strawberries.

T-minus two hours to Carb Party

To distract myself until Carb Party, I began making some homemade treats and within minutes, my spotless counter was cluttered with mixing bowls, flour, chocolate chips, sugar, bananas, Rice Krispies, marshmallows, cupcake icing, and M&Ms.

T-minus 30 minutes to Carb Party

I hit the door with my crumpled Carb Party wish list and my oversized duffel bag stuffed with treats.

While I sat waiting at the fast-food drive-thru I sent the following group text message to Laura, Natasha, Darnell, Jude, Donna and Mitch: "I'm getting waffle fries . . . does anyone need anything?"

T-minus two minutes to Carb Party (4:58 p.m.)

I arrived two minutes early and rang the doorbell.

My friend Natasha opened the door and greeted me with, "Wow, you're looking skinny!"

Once inside, I was smacked in the nose with the wafting aroma of warm brownies, cinnamon rolls, and fresh-baked chocolate chip cookies.

I walked into the kitchen and yelled my usual greeting, "Who's ready to kill some carbs?"

Within 15-20 minutes I manage to scarf down a handful of snickerdoodle cookies, two large homemade Rice Krispies treats, a slice of pizza and a bottle of kombucha. The sugar rush made my teeth tingle. I'm noticeably Carb Tipsy. I look around and see everyone moving from treat to treat filling up their plates with brownies, donuts, cinnamon rolls, and pizza.

Within 30 minutes I'm Carb Drunk and passed out on the couch.

I can't wait to do this again in six days!

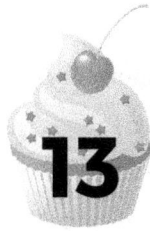

13

. . . .

52 Carb Party Ideas

Theme Parties

- **Mix & Match** – This is our #1 recommended party. This party will resemble a college dorm during finals week. Everyone brings the foods they've craved all week. The idea is to indulge yourself with everything on your "carb wish list." A wide range of sweet to savory treats will flood the kitchen countertops. Expect a variety of foods: pizza, Chinese takeout, Oreos, homemade brownies, hard candy, Cool Whip, chocolate chip ice cream, soda, and homemade Rice Krispies treats. With this party you'll be well on your way to losing 15 instead of gaining the "freshman 15"! #MixAndMatch

- **"Girls' Night Out"** – You've worked hard all week with career, kids and husbands, and school, and you deserve a night out on the town with your girlfriends. Imagine hanging out on a cool outdoor patio listening to live music and catching up on all your friends' funny stories. Laughter is good medicine, but be careful, you could overdose. After a few margaritas and funny stories, you'll be in fits of side-splitting laughter before the first bowl of chips and queso arrives. #GirlsNightOut

- **Gourmet Cupcake Party** – Turn on the TV to "Cupcake Wars" while you and your girlfriends embark on a friendly cupcake battle of your own. Your cupcake toppings and cake batter can be as tame or as wild as your imagination: crumbled bacon, candy sprinkles, toasted coconut flakes, orange zest, chili flakes, honey pistachio, s'mores, Butterfinger cupcake, angel food, peaches 'n cream, maple bacon, vanilla lavender, orange crème, PB & J, caramel cashew, spicy double dark chocolate, vanilla rum, or pink grapefruit.

  As an alternative to hosting a cupcake party, have a girls' night out at a bakery that sells gourmet cupcakes (e.g., Sprinkles Cupcakes in Dallas). #GourmetCupcake

- **Wine, Cheese and Chocolate Party** – BYOB! All week you've had to deal with whiney people. Wine'd down and toast your patience for annoying people with a glass of wine (or two). Imagine laughing with your girlfriends over glasses of wine paired with a variety of chocolate and cheeses from all over the world. Cheers! #WineCheeseChocolate

- **Progressive Dinner Party** – It's not the destination; it's the journey. Grab your favorite mix tape to jam to between restaurant stops. Start out with chips and queso (cheese) at your favorite outdoor patio and end the night with an after-dinner drink and crème brûlée at your favorite dessert spot. In the hours in between, plan on enjoying live music, dancing or even karaoke. #ProgressiveDinner

- **Gourmet S'mores Party** – These aren't your generic, humdrum, rinky-dink s'mores of your youth. These s'mores are red carpet-worthy. Plan to splurge on upgraded and exotic ingredients such as: dark chocolate, flavored marshmallows, sea salt caramel, Nutella, cookie spread, peanut butter cups, toasted coconut flakes, waffle cone crisps, chocolate graham crackers, and shortbread cookies. Envision your girlfriends gathered around a backyard fire pit or giggling around a living room fireplace. Remember, real friends will let you know if you have marshmallow smeared on your face before snapping that #CarbPartySelfie. #Smores

- **Gourmet Brownie Party** – This is the #1 Carb Party in Colorado, California and Washington. For some reason, regardless of careful planning, there never seems to be enough treats. LOL! This is an opportunity to get creative and not settle for the typical boring brownie. Go crazy. Get nuts. Go bananas. Add toffee, sea salt caramel, nuts, dark chocolate, peanut butter, fudge, M&Ms, pretzels, marshmallows, banana, butterscotch chips, or chocolate chips. #Brownie

- **Homemade Cookie Party** – An excuse to break out Grandma's famous cookie recipe. Finally an opportunity to eat your family's coveted "secret cookie recipe" without being forced to make small talk during the holidays with your creepy uncle. My family favorite is oatmeal chocolate chip, but perhaps yours is baklava, thumbprints, macaroons, sugar cookies, ginger snaps, molasses, snickerdoodle, oatmeal raisin or good old-fashioned chocolate chip. #Cookies

- **Breakfast for Dinner Party** – Come dressed in your PJs and slippers for the most important meal of the day: Carb Party! Let's be honest: For the past six consecutive days, breakfast has been pretty dull. You long for the sights and smells of breakfasts past. Your insulin practically spikes imagining fresh baked cinnamon rolls drizzled with icing, pancakes drowning in maple syrup, blueberry blintzes dusted with powdered sugar, Nutella-stuffed crepes, blueberry Greek yogurt topped with granola, cinnamon swirled French toast, jalapeno kolaches, and waffles piled high with fresh strawberries and whipped cream. Of course, no brunch is complete without mimosas! #Breakfast

- **Donut Party** – You've exercised self-control and resisted the office break room donuts all week long. Congratulations. This is your way of saying "in your face" to low-carb dieting while stuffing a few into your own.

Hannah: Laura, here's your chance to let your donut-freak flag fly!

Laura: Honestly, I feel like you haven't given donuts a fair shake.

Hannah: Believe me, I have. It's just that most people past the age of ten have evolved past their donut obsession.

Laura: Well that's depressing. A world without donuts isn't a world worth living.

Enjoy the "classics" like plain glazed, chocolate glazed, or go "fancy" with a variety of gourmet donuts like the blueberry-vanilla, Fruity Pebbles, peanut butter bacon banana, chocolate espresso, coconut vanilla bean, or habanero passion fruit. #Donuts

• **Fresh Baked Scone Tea Party** – This is your excuse to break out the dusty wedding gift tea set and try out your best fake English accent. Wear a ridiculously large hat to a table decorated like an English garden while enjoying warm scones and hot tea. #Tea

• **Retro Candy Party** – Travel back in time when cell phones were simply two tin cans connected with string. A time when your biggest "kid problem" was avoiding your family station wagon's backseat hump. BYOC (Bring Your Own Candy) while watching a retro movie like *Back to the Future* or *13 Going on 30* in beanbag chairs. Some retro candy: Zotz, Bit-O-Honey, Whoppers, Mike and Ike, Sugar Daddy, Hot Tamales, Milk Duds, Red Hots, Razzles, Pop Rocks, Fun Dip, Sky Bar, Bazooka bubble gum, M&Ms, $100,000 Bar, Twix, KitKat, Charleston Chew, Wonka Bar, Crunch Bar, Mr. Goodbar, Krackel, Dots, Warheads, Laffy Taffy, Airheads, Now & Laters, Raisinets, Ring Pops,

Lollipops, Tootsie Rolls, Life Savers, Chuckles, Neccos. #Candy

- **Pie Party** – Single ladies, all you single ladies . . . you finally have a good reason to make an entire pie. (**Laura:** I've eaten an entire pie and it's not easy!) You wanted to make a cookie dough cheesecake brownie pie or were curious what rhubarb pie tastes like. Now's your chance! Of course, who can think of pie without thinking of a pie-eating contest? So, ladies, make sure your pie isn't an epic fail—otherwise your door prize could be a pie to the face. Ready. Set. Bake! #PieParty

- **Kids Breakfast Party** – Remember having to fight with your brother or sister over who gets the "good cereal" in a variety pack? Guess what? At this party you won't have to call dibs on your favorite kids' cereal. Each Carb Partier brings a fresh box of their favorite: Lucky Charms, Cap'n Crunch, Reese's Puffs, Cinnamon Toast Crunch, Apple Jacks, Corn Pops, Cookie Crunch, Trix, Frosted Mini-Wheats, Frosted Flakes, Cocoa Krispies, or Honey Smacks. This is your time to reclaim all those tasty pastries marketed to kids in the following fun flavors: hot fudge sundae, s'mores, gingerbread, dulce de leche, ice cream sandwich, cookies 'n cream, chocolate chip cookie dough, chocolate fudge, confetti cupcake, strawberry, and brown sugar cinnamon. Why should the kids have all the fun? *CP Bonus: This is the only Carb Party that includes a toy! #Cereal

- **Disney Theme Party** – *Let It Go* and enjoy a Disney-inspired Carb Party. Test your knowledge with a fun game of Disney Movie Trivia while enjoying treats that are inspired by Disney themes and characters. Nosh on spaghetti as a nod to the classic *Lady and the Tramp* while sipping a homemade peach Bellini (or any adult frozen drink) in honor of *Frozen*. Some fun treat ideas are Rice Krispies snow balls (*Frozen*), caramel apples (*Snow White*), Oreo cookies and cookies 'n cream ice cream (*101 Dalmatians*), peanut butter cookies (*Dumbo*), homemade banana nut bread (*Jungle Book*), Hershey's Kisses (*Sleeping Beauty*), grilled pineapple skewers (*Leo & Stitch*), Swedish Fish (*Finding Nemo*), fruit chews, and Italian gelato (*Chronicles of Narnia*). Or perhaps you've waited all week for something starchy and exotic like jasmine rice (*Aladdin*). Just make sure your party wraps up before the stroke of midnight or else your car will turn into a pumpkin and you'll have to call a cab (*Cinderella*). #Disney #Frozen

- **Breast Cancer Awareness Party** – Where else can you show support by lounging around in head-to-toe pink while enjoying all your favorite pink-colored foods with your closest friends? Show your support for a good cause by wearing a pink feather boa and eating all things pink: cupcakes, Starburst candy, jelly beans, cherries, Popsicles, strawberry ice cream, pink-iced cookies, strawberry and banana smoothies, and pink M&Ms. #SaveTheTatas

- **Movie Night Party** – With the advent of digital streaming movies, the only thing missing now is the concession stand treats. Enjoy your favorite rom-com or award-winning indie film while eating all your favorite concession stand treats without the disgruntled employee attitude or the outrageous price tag. Place a bowl of freshly popped popcorn in your lap and a soda within arm's reach. If you're feeling a bit adventurous, try adding a box of M&Ms or Milk Duds to your warm popcorn. If savory is your thing, then make some nachos with jalapenos using real cheese. Some other movie theater treats include: Hot Tamales, Junior Mints, Sour Patch Kids, chocolate-covered almonds, Butterfingers, and SweeTarts. *CP Bonus: Never missing half the movie waiting in a long line to use the women's room. #Movie*

- **Duck Dynasty Party** – Dress code: fake beards and bandanas. Party décor: ducks and everything camo—paper plates, paper napkins, tablecloth. Entertainment: binge-watch a marathon session of Duck Dynasty while chowing down on the following Southern home cook'n: fried chicken, fried okra, mashed taters, fried pickles, green beans, sweet corn and creamed corn. Wash it all down with sweet tea from mason jars. Desserts include homemade blueberry cobbler, apple pie, and pecan pie. #DuckDynasty

- **Pool Party** – We strategically placed this Carb Party toward the middle to give your previous Carb Parties a chance to work. Now's the time to flaunt your new and improved bikini body. Girl, you're looking hot! The poolside grill won't be the only thing sizzling . . . cool down with frozen drinks, margaritas, Popsicles, Jell-O shots, fudge bars, ice cream sandwiches. #PoolParty

- **Academy Awards Watch Party** – Roll out the red carpet for a star-studded evening with your girlfriends to watch the Oscars. Celebrate celebrities and carbs. Tonight, everybody is a winner! The only real losers are your fat cells. Here's a fun drinking game idea: Every time a celebrity is asked, "Who are you wearing?" you and your girlfriends have to take a shot or (nondrinkers) eat another treat. Question: Which one of your girlfriends will be the one to take a chance, betting on Leonardo DiCaprio to win an Oscar? #AcademyAwards

- **Super Bowl Party** – If your Super Bowl contains broccoli or brussels sprouts, expect a flag on the play and a 20-yard penalty. Get your game face on and represent your favorite team by wearing your team's NFL jersey. Don't drop the ball— make sure there are enough chips, cheese, nachos, beer, craft beer, chicken skewers, dip, BBQ, jalapeño poppers, brownies, cookies, and Doritos for all four quarters. You may need a time-out to huddle up with girlfriends and decide what to eat next. Watch all the funny commercials. #SuperBowl

- **Little Debbie and Hostess Theme Party** – Debbie was your best friend growing up . . . she went everywhere you did. She went to elementary school in your lunch box and into the living room to watch TV. Celebrate all your favorite childhood snack cakes with this sweet-nostalgic Carb Party. Let your inner child roam free as you enjoy a variety of Little Debbie and Hostess Snack Cakes such as Zebra Cakes, Nutty Bars, Swiss Rolls, Oatmeal Crème Pies, chocolate cupcakes, Star Crunch, Honey Buns, Twinkies, Fruit Pies, Zingers, Ho Hos, Sno Balls, and Chocolate Frosted and Powdered Sugar Donettes. #Twinkie #HoneyBun

- **NASCAR Party** – It's hard to believe that America's #1 sport involves watching cars drive in repetitive circles— but statistics don't lie. NASCAR draws more viewers than any other professional sport including the NFL, NBA and NHL. We think it must have something to do with all the delicious infield tailgate food. Wear something comfy and enjoy a savory casserole, beer chili stew, triple-baked potatoes, and grilled kabobs, and wash it all down with your favorite chilled wine cooler or beer. #NASCAR

- **Board Game Party** – Take a Risk and get together for a night of board games. If you know anything about Carb Parties, your success is directly related to your Carb Sobriety. Therefore, we suggest competitive games start before you've had a handful of gummy bears, peppermint patties, and a few homemade brownies. Otherwise you'll be too Carb Drunk to win. The ideal atmosphere is when everyone is just Carb Tipsy. That way, everyone is hilariously uninhibited playing Charades but not yet crumpled in a corner in a Carb Coma. Some fun game suggestions: Jenga, Twister,

Pictionary, Taboo, and Cranium. *CP Tip: trivia game + Jell-O shots = Carb Party! #BoardGames

- **Lip Sync Battle Party** – You've logged hundreds of hours singing in the shower and in your car. Now it's time to throw down for a fake sing-off. Who doesn't want to see their most conservative Carb Party friend lip sync Katie Perry's *Last Friday Night* or Madonna's *Like a Virgin?* Win or lose, everyone is sure to get a laugh. If you need inspiration, watch Jimmy Fallon battle it out on TV with other celebrities. #LipSync

- **Dog Lovers Party** – It's been a *ruff* week. Meet your friends at your favorite dog-friendly *spot* and enjoy all your favorite foods. Today, enjoy your favorite carb knowing that its *bark* is worse than its *bite*. You deserve a party that's *paws*itively *off the leash*! Trust me, your friends will *beg* you to do it again next week. #Dog

- **Cat Lady Party** – This is the *purrr*fect Party for cat lovers be*claws* it combines cats and carbs. All week you've been saying, "If I have to go without carbs one more day, it'll freak *meowt!*" Get *frisky* and arrive wearing your favorite cat T-shirt. #Cat

- **Dance Party** – *So, You Think You Can Dance?* Then crank up the volume and get ready to shake your groove thaaannng. It's time to transform your living room into a dance floor. Showcase your best moves: Robot, Sprinkler, Super Man, the Running Man, Hoedown, Throw Down, Moonwalk,

Cabbage Patch, Electric Slide, Tootsie Roll, Vogue, the Wop, the Kid 'N Play, Harlem Shake, Krumping, Soulja Boy, and the Wobble. If you'd rather break out your own signature moves, then by all means, *bring it*! #Dance

- **Girl Scout Cookie Party** – In years past, you successfully dodged the cookie order form in the office break room. Unfortunately, your luck's run out and you're now the proud owner of seven boxes of Thin Mints. Repurpose your Girl Scout inventory along with your favorite store-bought cookies. Flavors include: Thin Mints, Caramel deLites, Peanut Butter Patties, Short Bread, Do-si-dos, Cranberry Citrus Crisps, Lemonades, Rah-Rah Raisins, Savannah Smiles, Thanks-a-Lots, Toffee-tastic, Trios. *Party drink*: Earn your drinking badge by serving a "Dirty Girl Scout" consisting of Bailey's Irish Cream, crème de menthe, and Kahlua. #GirlScoutCookies

- **Protein Bar Party** – Lest you forget, protein bars are essentially candy with added protein. If you don't believe us, look at the nutrition labels. On average, a protein bar has approximately the same amount of carbs as three store-bought cookies. Protein bars come in a variety of flavors including cranberry orange, green tea, honey, dark chocolate cherry almond, s'mores, peanut butter & chocolate, mint chocolate chip, double chocolate chunk, cinnamon, lemon, cookies 'n cream, apple pie, white chocolate raspberry, banana nut muffin, cinnamon roll, coconut cashew, peanut butter

& jelly. *CP Tip: Chop and serve with frilly toothpicks and complementary fruit smoothies. #ProteinBar

- **Ice Cream Sundae Party** – This is the ice cream lover's ultimate fantasy. If a candy store and an ice cream factory had a baby, you'd get this Carb Party. Let your flavor imagination run wild with an endless variety of ice cream sundae toppings: gummy bears, Reese's Pieces, hot fudge, fresh fruit, nuts, cherries, marshmallows, Fruity Pebbles, chopped almonds, chocolate chips, espresso beans, crushed graham crackers, M&Ms, candy sprinkles, toasted coconut flakes, crushed Oreos, brownie bites, and caramel sauce. *CP Tip: Top ice cream with your favorite liqueur like Kahlua or Drambuie. I scream, you scream, we *all* scream for ice cream! #IceCream

- **Fruit Bowl Party** – In this party, there's no such thing as "Forbidden Fruit." Go wild and try all those exotic fruits in your grocery store's produce department. Don't be a kumquat and go for the grapes. Reach for the *star* fruit: Grapple (apple-grape hybrid), some papayas, dates, jackfruit, goji berries, gooseberries, lychee, camu camu berries, pomegranates, and mangosteens. This is also a good time to try fruit in all its forms: freeze-dried, dried, fresh, or frozen. #Fruit

- **Craft Beer Party** – Engage in *flights* of fancy by trying all the obscure beers to be called a Certified Beer Snob. Pair your beer selection with various savory carb treats such as cheeses, brats, burgers, BBQ, and meatballs. Have fun with "liquid bread." #Beer

- **Tipsy Doodle Party** – What kind of art do you get when you finally eat sugar and drink a few glasses of wine? We're not sure if it has a name, but it looks sort of a like a juice box spilled on a Jackson Pollock painting. Beauty is in the eyes of the beholder. And at the end of this party, we guarantee those eyes will be blurry. #Doodle

- **Starbucks Party** – You've waited all week for your favorite coffee drink and sweets. With reckless abandon, you can order that Trenta Caramel Mocha Frappuccino with java chips, extra whip, and extra caramel drizzle. This is the only Starbucks meeting where "business talk" is prohibited and pastry display discussions are encouraged. So put up your laptops, and enjoy tasty treats in the company of your Carb Party friends. #Starbucks

Culture & Cuisine Parties

- **New Orleans Dinner Party** (Nawlins) – Who dat? Celebrate Mardi Gras without having to do something you'll regret. In other words, BYOB (Bring Your Own Beads). New Orleans is world-renowned for its delicious Cajun foods such as po' boys, jambalaya, red beans and rice, frog legs, crawfish, corn bread, bread pudding, pecan pralines, spicy boiled peanuts, muffalettas, crab cakes, and beignets. Transform your suburban living room into the French Quarter with a few fleurs-de-lis, jazz music and bottomless homemade Hurricanes. #NOLA

- **Asian Dinner Party** – Greet your guests in a Kimono (or budget-friendly bathrobe). Decor should include some of the following: Japanese lanterns, bamboo, fountains, goldfish (Goldfish crackers), and oversized stuffed panda bears. Enjoy snacking on stir-fried veggies, egg rolls, crab wontons, long grain white rice, fried rice, jasmine rice, sticky rice, and fortune cookies served from Chinese take-out boxes. Break out the chopsticks and pour some Saki shots. Desserts include: green tea ice cream, coconut ice cream, fried bananas, mango ice cream, and fresh oranges. If you prefer, meet your girlfriends at your favorite sushi bar and enjoy the tasty food presentation of a master sushi chef. #Asian

- **German Dinner Party** – It's Oktoberfest, sans the lederhosen. Eat your favorite German foods like schnitzel, cream puffs, pretzels, spaetzle, Bavarian cream pie, and German chocolate cake (ice cream, cake, cookies). After a few steins of dark beer, gather your guests into a circle and begin doing the chicken dance. At the end of the evening, tell your guests "Gute Nacht." #Germany

- **Italian Dinner Party** – Decorate the serving table with a red and white checkered tablecloth with a wine bottle candleholder. Pour glasses of Chianti along with your other favorite red wines for your guests to prepare to unleash their inner pasta addicts. It's finally time to enjoy all your Italian favorites such as spaghetti with meatballs, lasagna, cannelloni, and fettuccini, served with sides of garlic bread, antipasto salad and bruschetta. Desserts include: tiramisu, cannoli, Italian wedding cake, and spumoni ice cream. Weather permitting, move the party outside with a glass of wine and a game of bocce ball. #Italy

- **Mexican Dinner Party** – Greet your friends at the door riding a burro and wearing a sombrero and a poncho. (The burro is optional.) Help your guests release a week of pent-up stress by taking turns whacking on a piñata blind-folded while your speakers blast Tejano music. Enjoy classic Mexican food such as street tacos, empanadas, tamales, enchiladas, quesadillas, and sopaipillas drizzled with honey. Sip on imported Mexican beer while snacking on tortilla chips and salsa. Decor should include some Virgin Mary candles found at any dollar store. #Mexico

- **Greek Dinner Party** – This ethnic dining party includes a complementary theme movie. Turn on *My Big Fat Greek Wedding* or *Mama Mia* while dining on gyros, Greek salad, grapes, tzatziki sauce, Greek appetizer pizzas, Greek yogurt, and various honey-based desserts including baklava. For a decidedly Greek atmosphere, request that your friends arrive in bedsheet togas and laurel leaf headbands. #Greece

- **French Dinner Party** – Ooh la la! An excuse to drink lots of good wine! Greet your guests with "bonjour" and a pencil mustache. Your living room is now old Paris. If you look just beyond the entertainment center, you'll see the famous Eiffel Tower (8x11 poster). Create a French atmosphere with lots of pink/black/white accessories, bowls of fruit, art easels, and French music. Enjoy France's delicious flaky, sweet, and savory foods including: French toast, croissants, cheese puffs, French bread, baguettes, fruit tarts, quiche, macaroons, soufflé, cream puffs, baked brie, French onion soup, crepes, silk pie, and, if on a budget, Hot Pockets. #France

- **Hawaiian Dinner Party** – Greet your guests wearing grass skirts, coconut bras, and flip-flops with a welcoming flower lei and direct them to the backyard where a fire pit and kiddie pool filled with sand await. Accessorize the Hawaiian theme with giant tissue flowers and complement the atmosphere with music by Don Ho or Israel Kamakawiwo'ole. Sip on fruity cocktail drinks while nibbling on teriyaki chicken skewers. Other island treats include: bacon-wrapped pineapple, fruit kabobs, mango salsa, pineapple cheese spread, banana boats, Hawaiian rolls, Hawaiian pizza (ham, cheese, and pineapple), sand dollar cookies, gumdrops, and tropical flower-shaped sugar cookies. *CP Tip: Hire fire dancers—just be sure your homeowners insurance is up to date. #Hawaiian

- **Sci-Fi Party** – This party is out of this world! Distribute tinfoil hats to shield your guests from any stressful workweek thoughts, which would prevent them from enjoying the Carb Party. Binge-watch your favorite sci-fi themed show such as Stargate SG-1, Fire Fly, Dr. Who, or any one of the Star Trek series—Enterprise, Next Gen, Voyager, Deep Space Nine, or TOS (The Original Series). Continue the sci-fi theme with treats such as Pop Rocks, Rock Candy, Moon Pies, Milky Way Bars, and sugar cookies in the shape of planets. Repurpose your kids' Styrofoam solar system science fair project into a game. See who can disassemble and reassemble the solar system the fastest. To rehydrate, sip on glow-in-the-dark cocktails. Test your sci-fi knowledge with a game of trivia. The winner gets to choose next week's Carb Party. #SciFi

Seasonal Holiday Parties

- **New Year's Party** – Switch from counting carbs to counting down the remaining seconds of the year. Make sure to have all the obligatory New Year's accoutrements like champagne, wine, hors d'oeuvres, cheese, crackers, and mixed nuts. Make anything fancier by chopping up into small pieces to be speared with a frilly toothpick and placed on a silver platter. (Starburst, brownies, candy bars, cake balls, and fresh fruit) #NewYear

- **Valentine's Day Party** – "Roses are red, violets are blue, I love carbs . . . how about you?" Decorate your party by incorporating heart shapes and the color red. Fall in love with your favorite treats all over again, like chocolate-dipped strawberries, message SweeTarts, heart-shaped Rice Krispies treats, red velvet cupcakes, strawberries and cream puppy chow, pink sugar cookies, cherry lollipops, chocolate truffles, and red M&Ms. Sip chocolate martinis or a glass of wine and watch rom-com movies like *Sleepless in Seattle, While You Were Sleeping, Valentine's Day, Never Been Kissed, 50 First Dates, Along Came Polly, My Best Friend's Wedding,* and the classic *When Harry Met Sally.* #ValentinesDay

- **St. Patrick's Day Party** – Leave this party with the luck of the Irish and a pot o' carbs. Offer your guests Irish Cream cupcakes, Lucky Charms trail mix, beer bread, and bread pudding with custard sauce. Decorate your party with a rainbow of colors. Set out bowls of gold chocolate coins, rainbow Skittles, Mike and Ike, Lucky Charms and Fruity Pebbles cereal. If you're in a savory mood, enjoy shepherd's pie and Irish potato cakes with a Guinness beer. Of course, no St. Paddy's Day party is complete without green Jell-O shots or a green-colored cocktail. #StPatricksDay

- **Easter Party** – You won't have to hunt for tasty treats. All your favorite Easter basket treats are counter high and in plain sight. Feast on pastel-colored candy and pastries such as vanilla bean cupcakes with strawberry buttercream frosting and lilac fondant. Get creative with your girlfriends and decorate hard-boiled eggs. Each guest takes home a small basket of decorated eggs to be eaten the following six days of no-carb eating. Another great party activity is to make graham cracker birdhouses with Peeps. #Easter

- **Fourth of July Party** – "Your friends are here . . . the sky is bright . . . let's celebrate the Fourth tonight!" This party has the biggest bang for the boom! Watch the sparks fly as you and your friends dig into all your favorite star-spangled savory & sweet treats: burgers, beer, chili, ribs, corn on the cob, kettle corn, watermelon, blueberries, strawberries, ice cream, Pop Rocks, red and blue Jell-O shots, ice cream sandwiches, sugar cookies, brownies, cake pops, slushies, snow cones, apple pie, and blueberry pie. Suggested party games: beer pong, horseshoes, and beanbag toss. Wear your Daisy Dukes with your cowboy boots and flaunt your Carb Party body tonight! #4thOfJuly

- **Trick or Treat Party** – No tricks, only TREATS. You won't find those crappy "treats" that haunted you in your childhood like Halloween pretzels, fresh oranges, and black pencils. Only the best treats are showcased at this party: kid candies, miniature candy bars, SweeTarts, Tootsie Pops, trail mix, candy corn, orange punch, brownies, and popcorn balls. Feature spider and ghost decor, watch scary movies (*SAW*, *Friday the 13th*, *Ghost Busters*, black and white classics like *Dracula*), bob for apples, have a dipping station to make gourmet pretzels, and hold a pumpkin carving contest. #Halloween

- **Thanksgiving Party** – Leaf your worries behind and gobble until you wobble! Don't be a turkey—save room for the cornucopia of desserts that give you another reason to be thankful. You'll want to wear the proper gear (elastic waistband pants and oversized T-shirt) to comfortably enjoy the following: turkey-shaped sugar cookies, mini caramel apples on a stick (apple pops), mini cherry pie pops, pumpkin pie, pecan pie, Reese's Pieces, apple dumplings, harvest trail mix, candy corn, Chex mix, pumpkin bread, banana nut bread, chocolate pie, blueberry pie. Party drinks: pumpkin-spiced coffee drinks and cocktails. #Thanksgiving

- **Winter Wonderland Party** – We're making a carb list and checking it twice—you can party with us whether you're naughty or nice. Arrive dressed in your Ugly Christmas Sweater; it's a gingerbread house-making and cookie-eating party. You'll be drinking adult beverages during your gingerbread house construction, so there's no guarantee it'll be up to code. The following drinks are sure to warm your heart on a cold winter's night: hot toddies, spiked hot chocolate, wassail, spiked apple cider, Kahlua hot chocolate, snickerdoodle martinis, White Russians, peppermint hot chocolate, and eggnog.

Alternate Party Ideas: Holiday Movie Watch Party or White Elephant Gift Exchange. #Christmas

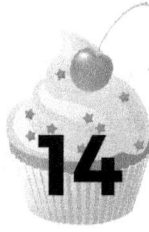

14

. . . .

Frequently Asked Questions

Q: Can vegetarians do the Carb Party Diet?

Yes, but it will be much more expensive than for carnivores. Since you won't be eating meat, you'll have to get your protein from protein powders. Most cheap protein powders have fillers and carbs. You will need to find a protein powder that contains less than five carbs per serving. Also, you'll need to supplement your dietary fat. A simple solution is to add heavy whipping cream or coconut oil to your shakes.

Q: Do I need to exercise?

NO! The Carb Party Diet will do 80% of the work without breaking a sweat. What you eat and when you eat will optimize your hormones to burn excess stored fat. Exercise if you like but your *main focus* should be on correcting your eating habits. Also, you won't be tempted to justify "falling off the wagon" by telling yourself "I'll just do 20,000 hours of cardio to make up for eating my entire Girl Scout cookie order." It's a lie. First of all, there aren't enough hours in the day to exercise away bad choices. Second, it only takes one cookie to raise your insulin and slam on the brakes of fat loss through a process called lipogenesis.

Q: What's the harm in eating just one cookie in between Carb Parties?

Again, it only takes one cookie, bowl of pasta or banana to elevate blood sugar levels. When your blood sugar rises, it causes a spike in your insulin. As a result, your body is signaled to store that sugar as fat through a process called lipogenesis.

Imagine asking for permission to eat just a little rat poison? " . . . but it's just a teaspoon of rat poison, what's the big deal? It's not like I'm pigging out on the stuff."

Your body doesn't give you "brownie points" (pardon the sugar pun) for doing the right thing most of the time. Sugar in any form will disrupt the fat-burning process.

So, you need to ask yourself if that one cookie is worth ruining your success between Carb Parties? You need to either be "all in" or "all out." Half-ass attempts won't give you the results you want and deserve. As Hannah and I like to joke: "Half-ass results lead to full-ass outcomes."

Q: Can 40-year-olds still lose weight with The Carb Party Diet?

Absolutely! Testimonials range from an athletic 21-year-old to a 34-year-old working mother of two, to a 48-year-old single mom.

Q: What is a Carb Party?

It's one designated night a week where you eat all your favorite carbs including cookies, cakes, and ice cream.

Q: Why do you need a Carb Party?

Your metabolism needs a weekly "one-night stand." (Don't worry, you won't have to do the walk of shame.) In other words, your metabolism begins to slow down after several successive days of eating a low-carb diet. Carbohydrate re-feeds (Carb Parties) trigger your fat-burning hormones to work at peak levels. Each Carb Party is like hitting a reset button on your metabolism so leptin levels are restored. As a result, your body is primed to burn stored fat at a much higher rate.

Q: What is a carb (carbohydrate)?

In short, carbohydrates are sugars and starches. A good way to easily identify a carb is to ask yourself if it is directly or indirectly derived from a plant. If the answer is "Yes," then it's probably a carbohydrate. Some examples of popular carbs are potatoes, rice, pasta, fruit drinks, honey, fruit, vegetables, flour, and candy.

Q: What is carb stripping?

Carb stripping refers to removing carbs from your diet. During this process, protein and fats should provide the majority of your calories.

Q: Why would any woman want to strip carbs from her diet?

Removing dietary carbs prevents insulin from spiking; as a result, your body is forced to burn fat as fuel in a process called lipolysis.

Q: Won't I feel perpetually hungry if my blood sugar is ultra-low?

Actually, when blood sugar remains ultra-low, so does your ghrelin, a hormone released in your stomach and intestines that communicates the feeling of hunger to your brain. When ghrelin levels are low, hunger pangs are low.

Q: What is insulin?

A hormone triggered by the ingestion of carbohydrates. Insulin's main job is to shuttle carbs (sugar) to your muscle cells, liver, or fat. Unfortunately, most overweight people don't place a daily demand on their muscles to use incoming carbs (i.e., sprinting, box jumping, weight training) and as a result, incoming carbs are stored as reserve fuel in the form of belly fat.

Q: Do I need to eat fat to burn stored fat?

Absolutely. Dietary fat is essential to mobilize and burn stored body fat. If you are dead set on eating lean cuts of meat, then we recommend you supplement your diet with the following types of fat: heavy whipping cream, butter, and cooking oil. Caution: Don't eat carbs with fat, as this macronutrient combo triggers the release of insulin.

Q: What is protein?

An animal-derived macronutrient. A quick and easy tip for identifying protein is to ask, "Did this food have a heartbeat?" If the answer is "Yes," it's either a protein or fat. If it walked, crawled or swam, it's probably a protein.

Q: Can certain food items have both protein and carbs?

Yes! Beware of foods that are processed with added sugar such as honey ham lunchmeat or breakfast sausage. Many BBQ rubs will also contain sugar, so read the ingredients on the nutrition label prior to using. In addition, protein bars are notorious for adding heaps of carbs in the way of rice flour, fruit juice, chocolate chips, and nuts.

Q: Can I use protein powder between Carb Parties?

Yes, if it's an ultra-low-carb protein powder mixed with water. Milk contains lactose which is a sugar and should be avoided. Please note: Protein powder alone can contain 1-12 carbs per scoop. The best alternative is to get your protein from whole meats, but if you choose to supplement with protein powder, make sure that you don't prepare it with milk.

Q: How can I eat low-carb at a restaurant?

Often, entrees will contain a combination of carbs and proteins (e.g., blackened chicken fettuccini). Obviously, the only Carb Party Diet "legal" part of this entrée is the chicken and Alfredo sauce. If the restaurant isn't too busy, kindly ask your server if the kitchen could hold the pasta and prepare a blackened chicken breast with a side of Alfredo sauce.

Q: How can I eat low-carb at a fast food restaurant?

Wrap your burger with large pieces of lettuce instead of buns. (Great for chicken sandwich, too!)

Q: How can I have a great Carb Party?

Keep a journal to track which party you did, who participated, and how you felt afterwards. Also, compile a carb wish list during the week. This is a great tool for coping with carb cravings during your six low-carb days and will serve as your Carb Party shopping list.

Q: How can I find others doing the Carb Party Diet?

Like/follow our Carb Party Diet Facebook page to make new friends and share Carb Party ideas like recipes, etc. Let's help each other!

Q: Is it possible to cut back to just one or two sodas and see results?

No! Soda is one of the leading contributors of obesity worldwide. It contains a sugar called fructose, which causes insulin resistance because of the way it's metabolized. Liver insulin resistance causes your pancreas to make more insulin just so the liver can do its job. Insulin then drives energy (calories) into fat.

Q: How will I feel during the first week stripping carbs from my diet?

Expect to feel a little sluggish and groggy as your body adjusts to burning fat for fuel. The mild side effects will subside within a few days. Your Carb Party is just six days away . . . you can do it!

Q: What can I snack on to help with cravings?

Sipping clear chicken broth throughout the day tends to curb cravings. You may also snack on nuts, deli meats, cheese sticks, and meat sticks. Later in the day, try decaffeinated coffee or flavored coffee beans (hazelnut, German chocolate cake, snickerdoodle, sea salt caramel, red velvet) with heavy whipping cream poured over ice. It's a refreshing alternative that tricks your brain into thinking it's getting a sweet treat.

Q: How can a carboholic like myself go without eating carbs?

Like any new challenge, your mental attitude will make or break you. To avoid any negative thoughts during the week, replace "I can't" with "I get to." It just takes getting through the first six and a half days until you "get to" have a Carb Party. Soon, you and your girlfriends will be enjoying fruit, bread, wine and all your other favorite carbs. So, don't give up!!

In addition, understanding the health consequences will help. Vanity issues aside, a carbohydrate-dense diet is unhealthy. The typical American diet is contributing to a worldwide diabetes epidemic. As an added bonus, you'll have fewer carbohydrates to feed bacteria on your teeth, which will lead to fresher breath and fewer cavities. You can do it!

Q: How will my sleep be affected?

On occasion, you'll dream of your favorite carby foods. You quite literally will experience "visions of sugarplums dancing in your head." Your unconscious mind will conjure up donuts, pastries, pizza, and other carby foods. These dreams can happen at any time but are almost guaranteed to surface within a day from your next Carb Party.

This scenario is the conscious equivalent of being stranded in the desert seeing a mirage, "Oh look, there's water," as you shovel handfuls of sand into your mouth.

Between Carb Parties, expect to have 3-D techno-color dreams of dessert trays piled high with chocolate cake, pastries, donuts or any other sugary treats.

Q: What's your craziest Carbmare? [Carb nightmare]

Hannah: My craziest Carbmare started something like this: I lifted the lid, peeled back the wax paper and saw a dozen warm, fresh donuts—glazed, chocolate glazed, sprinkles and even a cinnamon twist or two. Within seconds I killed the entire box! Then a second box . . . then a third. "It's OK if I go off the rails . . . I'll get back on track tomorrow," I thought. Dreams rarely make sense. Case in point, I dreamt about something that is full of gluten and I'm gluten-intolerant.

Q: Will the Carb Party Diet satisfy my out-of-control hunger?

After the first week of Carb Party, your appetite and cravings will decrease. You'll find yourself thinking, "Wow, I don't lick the plate anymore." Not because you're trying to be "good," but because of plummeting ghrelin levels due to carb stripping for six consistent days. (Ghrelin is a hormone that controls appetite.)

Q: When do you recommend shopping for Carb Party treats?

Don't Carb Party shop early in the week. Shop for carby foods close to the actual day of Carb Party or hide it in some obscure hiding place. It's too much of a temptation to have your favorite foods around while making a big change in the way you eat. Out of sight means out of mind.

Q: What can I drink during the week besides water?

Sparkling mineral water, diet sodas, iced tea, hot tea, coffee with heavy whipping cream (gin & vodka if mixed with plain water or soda water).

Q: What can't I eat during the week?

Avoid beer, mixed cocktails, bread, milk, rice, wheat, pasta, potato chips, legumes, beans, lentils, BBQ sauce, corn, processed foods, and salad dressings with sugar.

Q: Will I have to count calories?

No, your days of being obsessed with calorie counting are over; instead, you'll start viewing food as protein, fat and carbs. Your only concern now is whether or not the food you eat between Carb Parties contains carbohydrates. If the nutrition label shows it is zero or contains less than five grams per serving, then you eat it (i.e., cheese, meat, oils).

Q: Are foods labeled "No Added Sugar" allowed between Carb Parties?

BEWARE: No Added Sugar usually means "This product contains *carbs*"—usually in the form of fruit, oats, wheat, or nuts (i.e., protein bars, meal replacement powder, protein powder, and processed foods). This also includes all fruit which technically is "gluten-free," "all natural," and "no added sugar." A lot of times these already have 10-30 carbs per item. Don't get suckered by slick marketing.

Q: What's the difference between good carbs and bad carbs?

In regards to Carb Party treats, read the ingredient list and stay away from high fructose corn syrup and hydrogenated oils because they aren't good for your body.

Q: What did you do for your first Carb Party?

Laura: First Carb Party—I tend to go a little berserk with variety, trying everything. I used to have a treat hoarder mentality. I was like a squirrel stockpiling nuts in my cheeks to prepare for winter . . . but my "winter" was just six days away!

I'd freak out and eat a little of everything I couldn't eat during the first six days—all the "junk food" I wasn't allowed to eat during the week: ice cream, chocolate, waffles, peanut butter, Nutella, Popsicles. I over-indulged. My Carb Party prep included laying out all my treats in advance. Everything I dreamed of eating was at my fingertips. I wouldn't recommend doing it the way I did. I felt sick from overeating.

Q: How will I feel during my Carb Party?

You'll likely feel Carb Drunk from the sudden sugar high. If you're not drunk, you're going to be Carb Tipsy. You may fall asleep during a movie, but sleep will improve after the Carb Party . . . you'll fall asleep faster and rest deeper.

*CP Tip: "Friends don't let friends drive Carb Drunk." #Carbtipsy

Q: What can I expect the day after my Carb Party?

You may be a little bloated the day after the Carb Party and think, "Today I can't wait to eat carb-free!" (i.e., grilled chicken breast with broccoli). After several Carb Parties, don't be surprised if you have very little appetite at all the next day.

Q Have your cravings changed with the Carb Party Diet?

Laura: At the beginning of my Carb Party Diet journey, I ate a lot of treats that combined carbs + fat (i.e., ice cream, french fries, brownies, pizza). Now, after several months of doing the Carb Party Diet, I prefer straight carbohydrates. I used to crave super-sweet processed snacks and now I prefer fruit. Mangos, Fuji apples, apricots, and Craisins have replaced ice cream, potato chips, and candy bars. It wasn't a conscious decision to be "healthier" but rather the effects of removing sweets from my day-to-day life. To me, fruit is nature's candy. That's not to say if you offered me cookies or cake I wouldn't eat it. As a former Chocoholic, I still enjoy chocolate, but now it takes much less to be satisfied. I still eat whatever I want; it just so happens that I don't *crave* those things anymore.

Q: Which Carb Party would you recommend starting with?

I recommend the Mix & Match Carb Party as your first Carb Party. Enjoy everything you've been craving but couldn't eat, during that first Carb Party. To make sure you don't miss out and have any regrets, refer to a Carb Party wish list you compile during the week. My first Carb Party wish list looked something like this: ice cream sandwiches, Rice Krispies treats, chocolate wedges, Sour Patch Kids, gummy bears, Oreos, french fries, rice, chocolate chip cookies, mango sorbet, peppermint patties, homemade Brazilian cheese bread, chocolate covered almonds, and freeze-dried fruit.

Q: When should I weigh myself?

Never! Throw out your scale. The scale can be misleading. Rather, go by how you feel and how you look. Scales don't track fat percentages. You want your "weight loss" to be fat loss alone, not water loss or muscle wasting. A better way to track your progress is to take a "before" picture. So, throw away the scale, or at the very least, hide it—it messes with your head. Scales are flaky!

Q: When can I expect to see visible results?

Three to four days after your first Carb Party, you'll start to notice changes. However, results vary from person to person, based on starting body composition. Obviously, someone who is closer to an ideal body composition is going to notice a different level of success. In other words, it's more likely for someone who has a lower body fat percentage going into the Carb Party to say, "Wow, I can see my abs!"

Q: What are some of the hurdles we can expect doing the Carb Party Diet?

Expect people to not understand it. It's so counterintuitive because the world has been taught to eat a predominantly high-carb/low-fat diet. Also, the idea of purposely eating dessert one day a week sounds crazy to the uninformed.

Your friends will try to guilt you into eating carbs: "I made these cookies just for you!"

Q: How do I gracefully decline carbs from friends or coworkers?

Tell them you'll enjoy the treat later. "Later" in your case means during your scheduled Carb Party. Another tact is to tell them, "It hurts my stomach" or "It makes me sick." If you had a peanut allergy, they wouldn't force you to eat their homemade peanut brittle.

Q: Will I get tired of eating the same thing day after day?

Not any more or less than you did prior to starting the Carb Party Diet. Think about it, you were already eating the same thing day after day. You were probably eating the same two to three meats, but they were prepared in a variety of ways.

Therefore, experiment with a variety of spices to create a new experience using the same meats. Chicken can be prepared to taste as bland or savory as the spices you use.

Also, break the rules. Who says you can only eat traditional "breakfast foods" in the morning? Shake things up and enjoy that "hearty country breakfast" for dinner (i.e., scrambled eggs, sausage links, Canadian bacon, ham, and bacon).

Q: Can I financially afford to eat a carb-free diet?

Obviously, sugar and starches are cheaper than protein. That's why restaurants load your plate high with heaps of rice and noodles. Have you ever wondered why restaurants serve un-limited complimentary bread? Pound for pound, meat is more expensive. However, you can shop smart and buy in bulk at Sam's Club or Costco, or look for manager's specials.

Q Is it actually possible to save money on the Carb Party Diet?

Yes, it is completely possible. You'll stop impulsively throwing items into your cart because you'll shop from a planned shopping list. Also, you'll save by not buying the expensive prepackaged processed carbs. For example, a pound of chicken can cost less than one box of the most popular selling breakfast toaster pastries. Additionally, you'll stop going through fast-food drive-thrus and making late night, emotionally-driven ice cream purchases.

Q: What's a good tip to satisfy my sweet tooth between Carb Parties?

Trick yourself into thinking that you're having dessert by making low-carb (2-5 grams of carbs per serving) chocolate protein shakes with water and ice.

Kill the craving and move on.

Q: Is there any possibility of gaining anything during Carb Party?

Yes, but it won't be in the form of fat. What you'll gain is more discipline and self-confidence. Week to week, you'll be exercising more persistence and self-control. It's definitely a test—a test you'll *ace* with flying colors.

Q: Will eating fat make me fat?

The short answer is NO. It's a big fat lie that "eating fat makes you fat." It's eating fat combined with carbs that's problematic. Therefore, if you want to avoid getting fat, avoid eating fat combined with carbs between Carb Parties. (i.e., cake, bread and butter, pasta, pizza, french fries, pastries, casseroles, biscuits & gravy, mashed potatoes & gravy). Unfortunately, our brain chemistry is wired to *love* foods that are carbs + fat combos. When was the last time you wanted to curl up on the couch with a bowl of granulated sugar? That's right, never! Nothing heals a broken heart or crappy day at work better than our fatty-sugary favorites like chocolate ice cream, fresh baked cookies, brownies, fudge, and cupcakes. So go ahead, love the lard. Just make sure you shun the sugar.

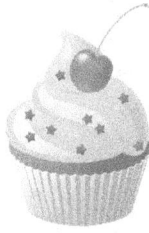

CHAPTER X

CONCLUSION

To be honest, we never intended to write a book. But after just a few weeks of bingeing on carbs, our friends and family started to notice. "You're looking great, what are you doing?" Our first instinct was to blurt out, "We do Carb Parties!"

Soon, our weekly Carb Party included a house full of friends and family. The next natural step was to share it with the rest of the world.

Laura: Let me explain something: I'm almost half a century old and I wear a size 4-6 jeans, regardless of whether I work out or not.

Hannah: And for me, it's all about enjoying bikini shopping. For years I've suffered PTSD from trying on my mom's too-tight swimsuit.

Laura: I'd be traumatized too if I had to wear my mom's swimsuit!

Hannah: Ha ha, Laura! I'm glad you can find amusement in my pain and suffering . . .

Laura: The best part is—we've lost all this weight and kept it off. I think it's because most "diets" require you to deny yourself something for the sake of losing weight and when you finally lose a little weight, you say, "Oh good, *now I can finally eat*." It becomes this yo-yo, swinging back and forth between deprivation and shame.

Hannah: Yeah, Carb Party is definitely a lifestyle. It's not something extreme that I'm doing to achieve a short-term goal with short-term results.

Laura: It's our "new normal." And I truly believe this will work for everyone. The only way it won't work is if someone gives up the first time they screw up. Truth is, nobody is perfect—otherwise our free will would be replaced with circuit boards. We're human not robots.

Let's be real. Between Carb Parties, you're going to have that slice of pizza (or three) in the office break room or a serving (or two) of your coworker's birthday cake, because heck—it's sort of weird to sing "Happy Birthday" with everyone and then sprint back to your desk empty handed.

Hannah: To be honest, even Laura and I have gone off track during the writing of this book . . .

I had just started doing Carb Party Diet when I got invited to WayForward Adventures, a charity organization that provides seven-day, guided, wilderness self-development trips. Rather than miss out on trekking around beautiful Colorado, I allowed myself to eat like the other girls on the trip: fruit, rice, beans, and candy.

Laura: And since we're all about being open and honest . . . I must confess, at some point during the writing of this book, I sort of had my own mid-life crisis.

I'm a 48-year-old, single, empty nester . . . need I say more? As if that wasn't tragic enough, (LOL!) I was suddenly laid off after 13 years with the same company.

How did I cope?

Well, I can assure you I didn't run out and buy a new red sports car.

Nope, I did what most women do regardless of age—I self-soothed on a never-ending supply of tasty carbs: ice cream, donuts, cookies, chips & salsa, pizza, candy, and frozen margaritas. For three consecutive weeks my pre-binge battle cry was *"I'm going out on a bang!"*

Hannah: Funny thing is—I think you actually believed it the first 20 times you said it!

Laura: More like 30 . . . but who's counting?

But you know what, it's OK! Life happens. The only things you'll ever do perfectly are the habits and lifestyle choices that packed on the pounds in the first place. That's because you've had 20, 30, 40 or more years of practice.

Matter of fact, I read it can take as long as 66 days to form a **new habit**. So—don't beat yourself up for momentary lapses and stumbles.

Hannah: I agree. When you have a less than perfect day—acknowledge it, get back on track, and move forward towards those motivational skinny jeans.

Laura: Right! The idea is when you fail—*fail forward*. Dust the cookie crumbs off your lap and get back on track quickly regardless of what day of the week it is.

Imagine that the process of losing weight is like navigating the Titanic. (Go with me for a second.) Had the captain made a tiny correction sooner, the Titanic would have missed hitting that iceberg and countless lives wouldn't have been lost. Don't wait until several days or weeks into a carb bender, before getting back on track. Lane changes are always easier than U-turns.

Hannah: And even if you follow the Carb Party Diet exactly, self-doubt will creep in and whisper, "Is this thing really working?"

One thing you *must* understand: reaching your weight-loss goals won't progress from one stage to another in a single series of predictable steps. Some weeks you'll lose weight and it will seem effortless. Your clothes will start to feel loose and you'll think "OMG, I'm melting!"

Laura: Later, you might feel "An acetylene torch couldn't melt this muffin top." The trick is to not quit.

Hannah: Actually, you *can* quit; this is a voluntary diet, not a cult! LOL!

Laura: That's right; you'll never be forced to drink the Kool-Aid unless it's sugar-free!

Hannah: But if you do quit and find yourself out of control— The Carb Party Diet is there for you. It's a quick, effective tool to get you back on track. You're only six short days away from getting your insulin levels back on track and enjoying carbs again.

Laura: The bottom line is—The Carb Party Diet worked for us and it can work for *you* too!

Hannah: Laura, it worked for you because I've agreed to be your daily donut slapper!

Laura: And that, Hannah, is why *I love you*! (And donuts!)

ACKNOWLEDGMENTS

From Laura

My future daughter-in-law, Hannah, without you none of this would be happening. I can't imagine doing this without you! Thank you so much for keeping me laughing and motivated throughout this past year. Also, I'm forever grateful you decided to date my son. Mitch may have found his future bride, but I found a lifelong friend and the daughter I never had.

Natasha Edwards, my carb-loving BFF, thank you for allowing your home to be Hannah's and my personal Carb Party playground every weekend for the past year! I (donut) you!

A million thanks to Chris Beattie, a truly gifted editor! Without your help, *The Carb Party Diet* would have looked like a five-year-old's pop-up book. Can't thank you enough! Denise Weldon-Siviy, a brilliant writer, thank you for all your expert help formatting and final editing.

To my McKinney, TX, peeps, Jude Parola, Toni Armeta Andrukatis, Michelle Stevens Bernard, and Lisa Titus-Page, thank you for your support and willingness to read rough, rough, rough drafts whenever ambushed in a restaurant, on the street, or anywhere else equally weird and inconvenient.

"Shout out" to my older sister Barb! It's about time I publicly acknowledged you for a lifetime of support. Good thing I wrote a book, huh? Thank you for being my #1 cheerleader, motivator, and stand-up comedy roadie.

Most of all, my son, Mitchell Sinclair—to say you were a constant source of encouragement would be a gross understatement. You simply wouldn't let me quit. And for that, I thank you.

From Hannah

Laura, the only thing more terrifying than writing a book is writing a book with your future mother-in-law. Well, actually, I take that back. The most terrifying thing would be writing a book with your future mother-in-law on an inflatable raft in the middle of the ocean encircled by hungry sharks. This is why I avoid large bodies of open water. All kidding aside . . . I love you! Seriously, I can't imagine a writing partner with more passion for helping people than you. You're not only my future mother-in-law, you're my partner in crime and best friend.

My future husband, Mitch, without you this book would not have happened. If it were not for you teaching me to eat like a man, I wouldn't have gone through my own personal transformation and been inspired to share it with the world. Thank you for encouraging me every step of the way—whether that was being a sounding board to bounce ideas off or listening to me talk about the book for hours on end. You truly are one of the most supportive people I know. (And the fact that you're good-looking doesn't hurt!) I can't express how grateful I am for you and I can't wait to start our life together.

Love, your future wife

ABOUT THE AUTHORS

Laura Bartlett is a donut-loving stand-up comedian in a family of doctors. She is the founder and executive producer of Four Funny Females, an award winning, all-female stand-up comedy troupe based in Dallas, Texas, created as a grass-roots movement to get women laughing again. In the same spirit, Laura taps into the power of "sisterhood" in her book The Carb Party Diet. She understands that anything is possible when women are helping women. To that end, she is thrilled to share a fat-loss solution that doesn't require women to restrict or remove themselves from meaningful social interactions for the sake of losing weight.

Laura began stand-up comedy at 36 years old, after delaying her comedy career to focus on raising her two sons as a single mom. She and her son Mitch are co-creators of the innovative bottle stopper called the Wine Condom, which has been featured all over the world, including NBC's Today Show, Meininger's Wine Business International, LA Times, and many more.

Hannah Sinclair is a former nationally-ranked high school women's wrestler who has spent most of her life as a human "diet" guinea pig. While her friends were trying to lose weight to look better in skinny jeans, she was trying to lose weight to pass the rigid weight-class requirements to remain eligible to compete. Her obsession with the bathroom scale led her down a path of experimentation with diet hacks and tricks that were ultimately damaging to her metabolism and overall health. Fortunately, she discovered a fat-loss process that is commonly known among elite male athletes but mostly unknown among women: the science of carb cycling. As a result, Hannah lost 15-20 lb. of fat while enjoying her favorite foods. Hannah now enjoys Carb Parties with her boyfriend, Mitch, and her Carb Party Diet co-author and future mother-in-law, Laura.

REFERENCES

Journal Articles

1. Margetic, S., Gazzola, C., Pegg, G. G. and Hill, R. A. "Leptin: a review of its peripheral actions and interactions," *Int. J. Obes. Relat. Metab. Disord.* 26, no. 11 (Nov, 2002): 1407-33. http://www.ncbi.nlm.nih.gov/pubmed/12439643

2. Allison, M. B. and Myers, M. G., Jr. "20 YEARS OF LEPTIN: Connecting leptin signaling to biological function," *J. Endocrinol.* 223 (Oct 1, 2014): T25-T35. http://joe.endocrinology-journals.org/content/223/1/T25.long

3. Friedman, J. M. and Halaas, J. L. "Leptin and the regulation of body weight in mammals," *Nature* 395 (22 October 1998): 763-770 | doi:10.1038/27376. http://www.nature.com/nature/journal/v395/n6704/full/395763a0.html

4. Wing, R. R., Sinha, M. K., Considine, R. V., Lang, W. and Caro, J. F. "Relationship between weight loss maintenance and changes in serum leptin levels," *Horm. Metab. Res.* 28, no. 12 (Dec, 1996): 698-703. http://www.ncbi.nlm.nih.gov/pubmed/9013745

5. Varela, L. and Horvath, T. L. "Leptin and insulin pathways in POMC and AgRP neurons that modulate energy balance and glucose homeostasis," *EMBO Rep.* 13, no. 12 (Dec, 2012): 1079-86. doi: 10.1038/embor.2012.174. http://www.ncbi.nlm.nih.gov/pubmed/23146889

6. Bernardo, A. P., Oliveira, J. C., Santos, O., Carvalho, M. J., Cabrita, A. and Rodrigues, A. "Insulin Resistance in Nondiabetic Peritoneal Dialysis Patients: Associations with Body Composition, Peritoneal Transport, and Peritoneal Glucose Absorption," *Clin. J. Am. Soc. Nephrol.* 10, no. 12 (Oct 27, 2015): 2205-12. doi: 10.2215/CJN.03170315. http://www.ncbi.nlm.nih.gov/pubmed/26507143

7. Yeo, W. K., Lessard, S. J., Chen, Z. P., Garnham, A. P., Burke, L. M., Rivas, D. A., Kemp, B. E. and Hawley, J. A. "Fat adaptation followed by carbohydrate restoration increases AMPK activity in skeletal muscle from trained humans," *J. Appl. Physiol.* (1985) 105, no. 5 (Nov, 2008): 1519-26. doi: 10.1152/japplphysiol.90540.2008. http://www.ncbi.nlm.nih.gov/pubmed/18801964

Terms and Definitions (in order of appearance)

Carbs: http://www.merriam-webster.com/dictionary/carbohydrate.

Dopamine: http://www.cbsnews.com/news/processed-carbohydrates-are-addictive-brain-study-suggests/.

FreshDirect: https://www.freshdirect.com/index.jsp.

Ghrelin: http://www.merriam-webster.com/medical/ghrelin.

Insulin resistance: http://www.ncbi.nlm.nih.gov/pubmed/26507143. See reference 6 above.

Lactose: https://en.wikipedia.org/wiki/Lactose.

Leptin: http://www.merriam-webster.com/dictionary/leptin.

Lipogenesis: https://en.wikipedia.org/wiki/Lipogenesis.

Lipolysis: https://en.wikipedia.org/wiki/Lipolysis.

Metabolism: http://www.merriam-webster.com/medical/metabolism.

Muffalettas: http://gonola.com/2012/08/24/muffaletta-mania-the-new-orleans-sandwichs-many-forms.html.

New habit: https://blogs.ucl.ac.uk/hbrc/2012/06/29/busting-the-21-days-habit-formation-myth/.

Obesity epidemic (official trailer for the movie Fed Up): https://www.youtube.com/watch?v=aCUbvOwwfWM. Also see http://fedupmovie.com/.

Programming your body to burn dietary fat and stored body fat as fuel: http://www.ncbi.nlm.nih.gov/pubmed/18801964. See reference 7 above.

Skip breakfast: http://fitness.mercola.com/sites/fitness/archive/2013/12/20/intermittent-fasting-weight-loss.aspx.

Spain's Seasonings: http://www.spainssmokehousespices.com/.

Sprinkles Cupcakes in Dallas: http://www.sprinkles.com/.

Strawberries and Cream Puppy Chow: http://www.justapinch.com/recipes/dessert/dessert-candy/valentine-s-day-strawberries-and-cream-puppy-chow.html.

Tankini: https://www.google.com/search?q=teenage+tankini+swimwear&rlz=1C5CHFA_enUS665US665&espv=2&biw=1419&bih=601&source=lnms&tbm=isch&sa=X&ved=0ah UKEwjFvIaw26HJAhVMOyYKHRTKA8YQ_AUIBygC.

Tramp stamp: http://onlineslangdictionary.com/meaning-definition-of/tramp-stamp.

Uber: https://uber.com/.

www.ingramcontent.com/pod-product-compliance
Lightning Source LLC
Chambersburg PA
CBHW060910280326
41934CB00007B/1267